fighting fighting
FAT FIT

Janette Marshall is an award-winning freelance author and journalist who specialises in researching and writing about food and health. A former deputy editor of *BBC Good Food Magazine* and editor of *BBC Good Health Magazine*, Janette is now a frequent contributor to many national magazines and newspapers and has had regular columns in both the *Independent* and the *Sunday Times*. Her previous books include: *Eat for Life* and *Healthy Eating on a Plate,* both published by Ebury Press.

Dr Mark Porter is one of Britain's best-known broadcasters on medical issues. After qualifying from Westminster Medical school in 1986, Mark started his television career on BBC1's *Good Morning with Anne and Nick*. Since then he has been a regular face on our screens, presenting a variety of health programmes including *Good Health* and *Morning Surgery*. Mark has recently joined BBC1's *Watchdog Healthcheck* team and is currently the resident doctor for both *Classic FM* and BBC Radio 2's *Jimmy Young Show*. A respected writer and journalist, Mark writes health columns for both the *Sunday Mirror* and the *Radio Times*.

Ainsley Harriott's larger-than-life personality has firmly established him as one of the nation's favourite tv chefs. First appearing on our screens as the resident chef of BBC1's *Good Morning with Anne and Nick*, Ainsley has since become one of the most popular contestants on *Ready Steady Cook* and *Can't Cook Won't Cook*. His summer cooking series, *Ainsley's Barbecue Bible* inspired a nation-wide wave of summer sizzling, while his most recent cookery series, *Ainsley's Meals in Minutes* perfected the art of tasty and healthy cooking in next to no time.

fighting fighting
FAT FIT

Eat Well – Get Active – Lose Weight

**Janette Marshall with Dr Mark Porter
and recipes from Ainsley Harriott**

This book is published to accompany the BBC Radio 2 and
BBC Education *Fighting Fat, Fighting Fit* health campaign which
was first broadcast in 1999.
Commissioning Executive for BBC Education: Fiona Pitcher
Senior Producer for BBC Radio 2: John Gurnett

Published by BBC Worldwide Limited, Woodlands, 80-Wood Lane,
London W12 OTT

First published 1999
Reprinted 1999, 2000

The recipes in this book first appeared in
In the Kitchen with Ainsley Harriott, *Ainsley Harriott's Barbecue Bible*,
and *Ainsley Harriott's Meals in Minutes*.

ISBN 0 563 38490 5

Commissioning Editor: Nicky Copeland
Project Editor: Rachel Brown
Copy Editor: Kelly Davis
Designer: Janet James

Printed and bound in Great Britain by Redwood Books, Trowbridge
Cover printed by Belmont Press Ltd, Northampton

A *Fighting Fat, Fighting Fit* video is also available
from BBC Worldwide
Catalogue number: BBCV6630

Contents

Introduction
Life is for Living (Not Dieting)
by Dr Mark Porter

The human body is an engineer's dream, a structure of unrivalled complexity that runs for decades with little or no maintenance. No wonder we tend to take it for granted. It's so reliable that we only truly appreciate it when it starts to go wrong, by which time it's often too late to undo the damage. I don't want to live for ever, but I do want to be happy and healthy for as long as possible so that I can live life to the full. That, in a nutshell, is what *Fighting Fat, Fighting Fit* is all about.

Think of your body as a car and yourself as the driver. Broadly speaking you can be divided into one of three types of owners. The fastidious *concours d'élégance* classic-car owner fettles and polishes his pride and joy every weekend but hardly ever drives it. The careless owner drives his car into the ground, never cleaning or servicing it, and complains furiously whenever it lets him down. The sensible owner lies in between these two extremes. He cherishes his investment and drives it sensibly, because he knows that if he looks after the car, it will look after him.

We don't need to be martyrs to our bodies – life's too short for that – but we shouldn't ignore them either. You don't need to know how everything works, or how to fix things when they go wrong – that's what doctors are for – but you should have a basic grasp of what you can do to help, and apply those principles whenever possible. Diet and lifestyle account for the lion's share of ill-health in the United Kingdom, and if you follow the basic steps in *Fighting Fat, Fighting Fit* I promise that you will reap major rewards for minimum effort.

You don't have to go the whole hog either. Any step in the right direction, however small, will help. This book contains no quick fixes and no fads, just sound basic information and tips that can be adjusted to fit your lifestyle. We want you to change it for the better – permanently. Sure you could shed a couple of stone on some ridiculously low calorie, ready-made diet, but while that may make you feel and look better in the short term it won't help in the long run.

The reason why book shops are full of quick-fix diet plans is that they don't work. Most are impossible to sustain for any length of time, and the minute you stop following them you go back to the eating habits and lifestyle that made you overweight in the first place. But instead of learning from your mistake, you go back and buy the next trendy quick fix, and so the cycle continues. The only people who benefit are those who write the books.

Fighting Fat, Fighting Fit is different. If you follow the tips it contains you won't need to buy any more diet books. You will have set out on the right road and shouldn't need to turn back. I have never been involved in a project like this before and, unless there is a sea change in medical understanding, may never do so again – this book has everything you need to know. Bad for future sales, but good for you! The BBC don't do this sort of thing very often, but when they do they invariably get it right.

So how have we done it? Well, to make the book easy to follow we have divided it into two sections. The first is designed to help you understand why eating habits and lifestyle are so important and identify what, if anything, you are doing wrong, and gives tips on how to improve matters. The second section is devoted to plans for healthy eating and a selection of Ainsley Harriott's delicious recipes which prove that the healthy option need not be the boring one – far from it.

Please don't go straight to the eating plans. To make the most of them you need to work out which one is most suitable for you. Completing the questionnaires in the first section will help you to identify the sorts of changes you need to make and point you towards the right plan. The *Fighting Fat, Fighting Fit* Slimming Plan has been put together to help those of you who need to lose weight. The *Fighting Fat, Fighting Fit* Maintenance Plan will help you stay at your target weight once you get there. The *Fighting Fat, Fighting Fit* Healthy Eating Plan is for those of you who want to adopt a healthier way of eating without losing weight.

But this is not just a book about healthy eating. Exercise is a vital part of any healthy lifestyle, and the plans all work best when they're used in conjunction with an increase in day-to-day activity. The questionnaires and charts in the first section help you to work out how active you are, and give tips on pain-free ways to introduce exercise to your life and improve your basic level of fitness.

You won't need a leotard. Improving your basic fitness doesn't have to involve joining a gym and spending hours on a step machine (my idea of purgatory). Far from it. We want you to do things that you enjoy and can easily manage, because if you don't enjoy them and can't fit them into your lifestyle you are unlikely to keep them up. Remember, *Fighting Fat, Fighting Fit* is all about making sustainable changes for the better, no matter how small.

To make matters more interesting we have included a number of celebrity contributions from my Radio Two colleagues – some more inspiring than others! How does Jimmy Young survive on just one meal a day? Suffice to say that I will be making sure *Fighting Fat, Fighting Fit* is available in the Broadcasting House library and the famous canteen.

I hope you enjoy the book and that it helps you live a long and happy life. Never forget that good health is just a means to an end. If you think about nothing else it can quickly become an obsession that interferes with your ability to make the most of life – or, to put it another way, it will make your life feel like an eternity whether you live longer or not. Moderation never killed anybody – having a little of what you fancy every now and then is what life is all about.

Dr Mark Porter MB BS DA DCH

★ ★

★ Let the flight from fatness begin!

'Many, many years ago, intoned the Old Geezer, when I was a Boy Broadcaster, and in the peak of physical condition, I initiated an exercise programme on BBC Radio One and Two. It was called 'Fight the Flab', and became enormously popular. Well, I liked it… but, then, I didn't actually participate in the exercises – couldn't, you see – be out of breath for the broadcasting…

'Anyway, now, by all that's holy, the BBC is at it again. God loves a trier – let the Flight From Fatness Begin!'

A popular member of the BBC Radio 2 broadcasting team, **TERRY WOGAN** is no newcomer to fitness campaigns, as he explains. He does, however, admit to being better suited to encouraging others than actually participating himself.

★ ★ ★ ★ ★ ★ ★ ★ ★ ★ ★ ★ ★ ★ ★   TERRY WOGAN

Presenter of BBC Radio 2's *Wake Up to Wogan*

Chapter 1

Weighty Problems — Why Are We Fat?

Something extraordinary has happened in the last 20 years. As a nation, we have gradually been eating fewer calories; yet, at the same time, more and more people have become overweight. Today more than half Britain's adults are overweight and one in five men and women are obese. If we carry on at this rate it is possible (though unlikely) that one in four adults will be obese by the year 2005 and the entire population will be obese by the year 2050!

And that probably includes today's dieters. Because, despite an estimated one in three women and one in five men being on a slimming diet at any one time, we keep getting heavier. It has been estimated that, as a population, we are putting on around 1 gram a day or nearly 400g (just under 1lb) per year.

But how can this be?

While our eating habits may have changed, the basic equation remains the same. If 'calories taken in' equal 'calories used' then normal weight is maintained. The problem is that, although we are eating less, we are also burning fewer calories. It only takes a small long-term imbalance between energy intake and expenditure to produce weight gain. For example, a daily small bar of chocolate (containing around 100 calories), in excess of needs, would result in a gain of 4kg (9lb) over a year.

Our sedentary lifestyle means that we don't burn off as many calories as we used to. We are simply not active enough. This doesn't mean there aren't enough athletes around – it just means we don't do enough each day. Cars, escalators, electric lawnmowers and other labour-saving devices mean we are physically far less active. It might seem as though we are rushing around doing a great deal. And, indeed, we probably achieve more than we used to. But it is no longer the 'norm' to carry heavy shopping, to cycle or walk to school or work, do heavy housework, dig the allotment or garden, mow the grass with a manual lawnmower or play football. Far fewer men do manual jobs. We go everywhere in cars, watch football on TV instead of playing it and spend more time sitting at computer screens. While we have tried to compensate for our lack of physical activity by eating less, we still eat more calories than we burn.

There are also far more opportunities to eat than there were 20 years ago. This has been attributed to the 'McDonaldization' of the world. There are fast-food outlets and convenience stores on virtually every high street, and confectionery shops on every street corner and railway platform. With fewer family meals being eaten at home, people often eat on the bus, tube, train and while walking along the street. The companies who market convenience food encourage us to 'graze' in this way, and get us used to the idea from the cradle by aiming snack food advertisements and sponsorship at infants, toddlers, children and adults. Food is increasingly a part of every activity. We are in danger, it seems, of becoming a nation of passive over-consumers.

Some anthropologists argue that we are genetically programmed to eat whenever we see food. Our natural instinct to feast at every opportunity was essential to our survival, when we first evolved millions of years ago, as food was scarce. We are therefore equipped with extremely efficient appetites that spur us on to find food even before we are really hungry (hunting down a herd of wildebeest took a lot longer than popping into a supermarket!). Stomachs growl with hunger or with habit and, like Winnie-the-Pooh, we seek out 'a little something' at regular intervals throughout the day. We even eat when we have no appetite – just the sight of food can make us want to eat. Unfairly, the mechanisms that switch off our appetite seem to be far less efficient than the ones that trigger it.

There are other factors, too, that conspire to undermine our best efforts not to put on weight. We are cajoled into eating more than we want by social convention, and by not wishing to offend family and friends. And we turn to food for comfort, to reward ourselves, and to combat stress.

Except for fruit and bread-based snacks, most convenience foods such as ready-made meals, processed foods, takeaways, confectionery and savoury snacks are high in calories and fat. The high fat content of these easily available foods is another reason why it is so easy today to put on weight.

Dietary fat is a particularly important factor in weight gain. In affluent countries, where a greater proportion of calories are eaten as fat, the problem of obesity increases. This is because fat in food is more readily turned into body fat than calories from other sources such as starchy foods (carbohydrates), vegetables, fruit and protein. Starchy foods, fruit and vegetables are also much bulkier to eat, making it harder to consume too much of them.

The problem about putting on weight is that, once you become seriously overweight, complex changes occur in the body, changing the speed at which you burn off calories and altering your appetite, making it extremely difficult to lose weight. Prevention is therefore definitely better than cure when it comes to weight problems.

Does being fat matter?

Despite the opinions of some overweight people who say they are victims of 'fat fascism', being overweight *does* matter. Obesity is the commonest cause of ill-health in the UK. It contributes to illness and death from heart disease, respiratory disease, diabetes, gallstones and some cancers. There are more heart attacks among obese men and women, particularly those under 50 years of age. And the risk goes up, the fatter you are.

Even if you aren't obese, just being overweight is associated with a range of health problems that, in themselves, increase your risk of heart disease: raised blood pressure, impaired glucose tolerance and raised

Snacking can help weight control

Snacking has often been blamed for passive over-consumption and obesity. Yet research has shown that people who snack a lot are no fatter than those who do not snack.

● One study compared the effect of four different types of snack – high-fat, low-fat, sweet and non-sweet. The subjects were encouraged to eat 25 per cent of their food as snacks, and their intakes of calories, protein, fat and starchy foods were measured, as well as changes in hunger, mood and appetite. After six months it became clear that those who ate low-fat snacks freely, ate nearly 100 calories per day less overall than when they ate other types of snacks or no snacks. If maintained over a year, this would result in weight loss of around 4kg (9lb).

● The other health benefit of eating low-fat snacks (sweet and/or savoury) was a 20 per cent reduction in total daily fat intake. Complete freedom to eat snacks did not cause noticeable over-eating. And the low-fat snackers reduced the total number of calories from fat in their diet from 37 per cent to 33 per cent – meeting healthy eating targets.

● This shows that nibbling may actually help you stick to dietary guidelines and be beneficial to appetite control and health; whereas gorging does seem to contribute to obesity. For snack suggestions, see snack list A (page 106), snack list B (page 107) and snack list C (page 113).

insulin levels (which lead to arterial damage), higher levels of harmful types of cholesterol in the blood and lower levels of protective types of cholesterol. Even constipation, haemorrhoids and dental decay occur more often in overweight people. It certainly is a heavy burden!

How do you shape up?

It's not just fatness *per se* that threatens good health. Your risk of heart disease also partly depends on how the fat is distributed in your body. Men and women who tend to become apple-shaped, with fat deposited around the tummy, are at greater risk than those whose excess fat is distributed about the hips and thighs, making them pear-shaped.

For all those disappointed slimmers who have tried to change their basic body shape through dieting: sorry! Whatever you have previously been led to believe, it is a physical impossibility. If you are basically a pear shape you cannot become an egg-timer shape through dieting. However, you can become a smaller, leaner, trimmer, firmer or more muscular pear shape by becoming more active and eating a well-balanced diet.

And drinking less alcohol will also help, especially if your alcohol consumption is in addition to normal calorie requirements. Alcohol cannot be stored in the body so we burn calories from alcohol instead of using fat. And when fat isn't being used for energy it is stored as body fat. Some experts think alcohol is more likely to enhance 'apple-shape' weight gain around the waist. And such central deposits of fat are associated with health risks such as heart disease and high blood pressure.

Avoiding fatty foods also helps. Strictly speaking, any food can be fattening if you eat more than you burn in your daily activities. But fat is most readily converted into body fat. For this reason, and other health reasons, it makes sense to limit your intake of fat and fatty foods.

Without wishing to get the problem of excess weight out of proportion, it does matter to a lot of people. And it matters especially to give children the benefit of a good start in life – with a love of good food, well-balanced eating habits and enjoyment of physical activities.

Myths about dieting

1. Fat people burn calories more slowly than slim people

For years scientists were deceived into believing that overweight people ate less than slim people, took more exercise and were victims of their energy efficiency. They thought fat people must burn calories more slowly than slim people. The deception was uncovered during a study of the actual amounts of food eaten by obese people. This revealed that fat people expended more energy than slim people, which meant they must be eating more than they said they ate. Overweight people typically underestimate their calorie intake by around 800 calories a day – the equivalent of a medium bar of chocolate plus a moderate chunk of cheese.

2. I can't lose weight – it's my genes

During the last 20 years there has been a major rise in excess weight and obesity, yet our genetic make-up has not changed. Fatness does run in families, but not usually because families share genes – the genes from two parents normally differ widely. The main reason that whole families tend to be overweight is that they share the same eating habits.

There is also little evidence, so far, that some 'families' in the global sense (of races or populations) are more susceptible to obesity for genetic reasons. On the whole, differences are caused by environmental factors such as diet and the amount of physical activity taken.

However, many researchers are trying to discover any genes that might predispose people to weight gain. For example, there is a lot of interest in leptin, a protein that travels from fat deposits to the brain, giving it information about how much fat the body has on deposit. Leptin then probably triggers chemical reactions that increase or suppress our intake of fat and influence how much more fat is deposited by the body. Obese people have high levels of leptin in their blood. This suggests that there may be faulty receptors in their brains so that the messages can't get through to help prevent the pounds piling on.

While genetics cannot be blamed at the moment for the spread of obesity there are genes associated with appetite control and so-called 'satiety responses' (messages received by the brain, when you have eaten enough, that lead you to feel full and stop eating). People affected might not feel full in the same way that normal-weight people do when they have eaten. However, there is no need for them to despair – they do not have to be 'victims' of their genes. The good news is that eating habits are largely learned and can be adjusted, and more physical activity can also help.

3. It's not my fault – I have a slow metabolic rate

Many overweight people think they must be different to other people or think they burn fewer calories or burn their calories more slowly. The rate at which you burn calories is called your metabolic rate and it varies throughout the day, depending on whether you are resting or active. Generally men need about 2500 calories a day and women need about 1900, although the young need more and the elderly need fewer calories. People who claim to have a slow metabolic rate usually turn out to have a normal metabolic rate when subjected to strict scientific scrutiny.

4. I was normal weight until I gave up smoking

Not everyone puts on weight when they stop smoking. When appetite, previously suppressed by smoking, recovers, it is normal to put on a few pounds. But this weight can be lost in a matter of months, once you are more comfortable and can make adjustments to food intake and physical activity. The main thing is to stay positive. If your appetite increases you probably won't have to eat less, just differently.

5. There's something wrong with my glands

Genuine medical conditions that cause weight gain are very rare. They include hypothyroidism, in which the thyroid gland does not produce enough thyroxine to keep the metabolic rate high enough. Symptoms include feeling cold, tired all the time, experiencing weight gain and constipation. See your GP if you suspect that you have thyroid problems.

Fluid retention can also show itself as an increase in weight. It may be cyclical (linked to the menstrual cycle) in women, and can cause bloating of the abdomen. Or it may be caused by medicinal drugs, including corticosteroids and oral contraceptives, or a more serious underlying problem such as heart or kidney disease. See your GP.

6. Everyone puts on weight as they get older

Weight gain with age is not inevitable. It is usually a consequence of continuing to eat the same amount while being less active. It can also be the result of consistently over-eating, even by just a small amount, over the years. For example only about 40 calories a day, the equivalent of a mini Danish pastry, more than you need can result in a weight gain of 2.25kg (5lb) in a year.

7. Chocolate is my downfall – I give it up, then I just binge on it

Self-denial is the surest way to put on weight. It works every time. There's nothing wrong with chocolate. The biggest problem, particularly for many women, is to admit that certain foods are not 'naughty', and to learn to enjoy them. The best way is to enjoy a little of something as soon as you feel like it. A small amount of high-quality chocolate is more enjoyable (and less fattening) than denial followed by a binge. All foods can be enjoyed as part of a well-balanced diet.

8. I never had a weight problem until I got married/ had a baby/ took on this stressful/boring job...

Many people blame their weight problems on an event or change in their lives which is really a normal occurrence that does not lead to weight gain in other people. They suddenly become fat during or after a particular life event. For example, it's quite possible to find that you eat more when you marry because you may be at home more often, sitting in front of the TV, or you may find yourself following a more structured routine with regular, bigger meals. Parenthood can disrupt eating habits and cause women to behave like dustbins – eating with the children, eating up all the leftovers, eating again with their partner. Both stress and boredom can lead to over-eating as a way of trying to calm or compensate feelings (they can also have the opposite effect). The key, in these circumstances, is to recognize the changes that are happening and seek help from a professional such as a dietitian, counsellor or psychotherapist.

Why diets don't work

There are some people who enjoy following the most bizarre crash diets. It can be an interesting pastime to survive on pineapples and baked beans, or grapefruit and boiled eggs, for a few weeks. It is a wonderful conversation topic and a great hobby! It gets rid of the pounds before a holiday, before a wedding, or before a job interview. But it's even better to get back to your old (eating) habits! The trouble with becoming a habitual dieter is that each time you try a new diet, the weight is more difficult to lose and the amount of weight gained between diets goes up. So, what's going wrong...?

Intermittent dieting (especially on crash or very low-calorie diets of between 600 and 800 to 1000 calories a day), followed by a return to poor eating habits or over-eating, causes weight to yo-yo. This sort of on-off dieting is actually more dangerous to health than being slightly overweight all the time. As many dieters know to their cost, crash diets cause the metabolic rate to drop in order to conserve energy as the body adapts to starvation conditions. Weight then tends to be regained more quickly as the body tries to replenish its energy stores – so dieters can end up heavier than before.

If a diet is not well balanced it can also leave you short of essential vitamins and minerals, putting you at risk of anaemia and other health problems. Diets that contain too little starchy food may force the body to burn its own protein (muscle) for energy, causing muscle wasting or even loss of heart muscle or damage to the kidneys.

How dieting can get out of control

Dieters do not use the body's natural controls – they do not eat when they are hungry and when suitable food is available. Because the body's natural appetite controls have been overridden, eating can easily get out of control once they do start to eat. This is a familiar scenario – when a dieter blows a diet he or she simply gives up, and ends up bingeing on 'fattening' foods.

Dieters often seem to go completely mad on fattening food immediately before they set a date to restart the diet. 'Forbidden foods' (those that dieters think they should not eat) are more likely to cause a breakdown in the diet. Under the stress of dieting they lose sight of the long-term goal and (as they see it) fall prey to the temptations of food.

All this has led some psychologists to conclude that diets are dangerous because dieters develop unhealthy attitudes towards food. In susceptible individuals the same attitudes, when taken to extremes, can develop into eating disorders. However, this is not to say that diets lead to eating disorders such as anorexia nervosa.

If dieting goes too far

Dieting is never risk-free, particularly for teenage girls who should be growing and are supposed to be getting heavier rather than lighter. Nowadays even pre-teens often have a fear of being overweight. They think they are far heavier and fatter than they actually are. In response to comments from boys and friends that they are fat or unattractive, or to their own desire to match the unhealthy and unrealistic thinness of fashion models, girls become highly 'restrained eaters' who frequently diet.

While believing they are asserting their independence by controlling what they eat through dieting, teenagers are giving in to media, peer and social pressure to conform to a particular appearance. Nobody knows how to prevent eating disorders. There is no hard evidence that any one approach works. But the earlier the problem is recognized and treated, the better. A good starting point is the family doctor because, in order to gain access to existing services, the condition has to be diagnosed.

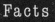

Facts

Good reasons why diets don't work

1 When you go on a diet your metabolic rate drops because your body adapts to starvation conditions by conserving energy.

2 Once you have lost weight, you need to continue to eat less than you did before in order to maintain the weight loss. So if your diet did not retrain your eating habits, you will regain the weight twice as quickly as you lost it.

3 Dieting also upsets your body's normal regulatory mechanisms for weight control. This often leads to over-eating.

4 Denying yourself particular foods sets up cravings that lead to over-eating or binge eating.

5 Restricting energy intake leaves dieters feeling lethargic so they are unlikely or unable to enjoy physical activity. Yet exercise is the best way to improve body shape and tone – the main aim of most dieters!

6 Dieting can lead to an obsession with food, making it very difficult to concentrate on work or anything else. This is why dieters may be slimmer but dimmer!

7 The stress of dieting may lead to depression and other emotional and behavioural problems.

Clearly, dieting creates a whole new set of difficulties and is not a solution to being overweight.

If dieting doesn't work, what does?

If you already have a weight problem, try not to gain any more weight. Try cutting down on food gradually by following the *Fighting Fat, Fighting Fit* Slimming Plan (see page 97). Then maintain your lower weight by following the healthy eating advice given throughout this book and the *Fighting Fat, Fighting Fit* Maintenance Plan (see page 136).

Gradual weight loss – an average of 1.5kg (2–3lb) a week – on the *Fighting Fat, Fighting Fit* Slimming Plan will result in *permanent* weight loss.

Don't forget the pleasure principle

Amid all this talk of weight problems and dieting, it is easy to overlook the pleasure principle. Remember to eat as widely as possible from the foods available to you. Enjoy a little of what you fancy, and give up any guilt complexes you associate with particular foods. Food is there to be enjoyed and excess weight can largely be controlled by following the old maxim – everything in moderation.

Now turn to Chapter 2 to see if you really do need to lose weight or if you just need to change some of your eating habits.

Do You Need to Change Your Eating Habits?

If you answer the questions on the following pages you can find out how many portions of food you eat from each of the main food groups per day. You can then compare what you eat now with the ideal intake for your age. The second part of the chapter shows how the amount of food you need changes according to your age, sex and level of activity. For example, older inactive women will need the lowest number of portions per day and younger active males the highest.

Your needs change not only throughout your life but virtually every day. Do not worry if you do not match the model on a daily or weekly basis or in particular areas. It is the long term that counts. The aim of this book is simply to get you started and help you do what you can – and enjoy what you do.

Portions

The amounts shown in brackets in the following lists represent one portion. In other words, 6 tablespoons of breakfast cereal is the equivalent of two portions (2 × 3 tablespoons). If you eat this amount in a normal day, write '2' in the space provided.

Eating Habits Questionnaire

1 How many portions of the following foods do you eat in a normal day?

Bread, potatoes, pasta and other cereals
.... breakfast cereal (3 tablespoons)
.... muesli (2 tablespoons)
.... bread or toast (1 slice)
.... pitta, naan or chapatti (1 small)
.... bread roll, bap or bun (1)
.... crackers or crispbreads (3)
.... potato (1 medium)
.... boiled rice (2 heaped tablespoons)
.... boiled pasta or noodles (3 heaped tablespoons)
.... plantain or sweet potato (1 medium)
━━━━━ TOTAL

Vegetables and fruit
.... vegetables or salad (1 medium helping)
.... fresh fruit (1 piece)
.... stewed or canned fruit (6 tablespoons – 140g/5oz)
.... fruit juice (1 small glass – 100ml/3½fl oz)
━━━━━ TOTAL

continued...

Milk and dairy produce

.... milk (1 medium glass – 200ml/⅓ pint)

.... Cheddar-type cheese (1 matchbox-sized piece –
40g/1½oz)

.... yoghurt, cottage cheese or fromage frais
(1 small pot – 125g/4½oz)

_____ **TOTAL**

Meat, fish and vegetarian alternatives

.... beef, pork, ham, lamb, liver, kidney, chicken
or oily fish (3 medium slices – 50–70g/2–3oz)

.... white fish, not fried in batter (115–150g/4–5oz)

.... fish fingers (3)

.... eggs (1)

.... Cheddar-type cheese (1 matchbox-sized piece –
40g/1½oz)

.... baked beans or other cooked pulses, lentils, dhal
(5 tablespoons – 200g/7oz)

.... nuts, peanut butter or other nut products
(2 tablespoons – 60g/2¼oz)

_____ **TOTAL**

Foods containing fat

.... margarine or butter (1 teaspoon)

.... low-fat spread (2 teaspoons)

.... cooking oil, fat or ghee (1 teaspoon)

continued...

.... vinaigrette (salad dressing) or mayonnaise
(1 tablespoon)

.... cream (1 tablespoon)

.... crisps or other savoury snack (1 packet)

.... other fatty foods, e.g. fried food, pastry, meat
products, sausages, pâtés, fatty bacon

_____ **TOTAL**

Foods containing sugar

.... sugar (1 tablespoon)

..............jam/honey (1 rounded teaspoon)

.... biscuits (2)

.... cake (1 slice) or a doughnut or Danish pastry

.... chocolate (1 small bar)

..............sweets (1 small tube or bag)

_____ **TOTAL**

Drinks (non-alcoholic)

.... coffee (1 cup or mug)

.... tea (1 cup or mug)

.... squash, fizzy drink, diet, slimline or sugar-free
drink (1 glass or can)

.... water (1 glass)

_____ **TOTAL**

continued...

Q

Alcoholic drinks

.... normal-strength beer or lager (300ml/½ pint)

.... wine (1 small glass – 125ml/4fl oz)

.... spirits (1 pub measure)

.... fortified wine, e.g. sherry, vermouth (1 pub measure)

_____ **TOTAL**

2 How do you match up?

Write your totals below:

.... bread, potatoes, pasta and other cereals

.... vegetables and fruit

.... milk and dairy produce

.... meat, fish, eggs and vegetarian alternatives

.... foods containing fats

.... foods containing sugar

.... drinks (non-alcoholic)

.... alcoholic drinks

continued...

3   What should you aim for, according to your age, sex and level of activity?

Bread, potatoes, pasta and other cereals

Write in your total number of portions per day (see opposite) and compare it with the recommended number for your age, sex and level of activity.

....

These foods provide you with the energy you need to be active and, in the case of younger people, to grow. They should be the main part of most meals and snacks.

Active women

Age	Portions per day
11–14	7–9
15–18	9–11
19–49	8–10

Sedentary women

Age	Portions per day
11–14	5–7
15–18	6–8
19–49	6–8

Women of 50+ 6–8 portions per day

Active men

Age	Portions per day
11–14	9–11
15–18	10–14
19–49	10–11

Sedentary men

Age	Portions per day
11–14	7–9
15–18	9–10
19–49	8–10

Men of 50–65 need 7–10 portions per day
Men of 65+ 6–8 portions per day

continued...

★ ★

★ ## Normal weekends – weeks out of kilter

'5am – I drive to work and take a piece of fruit to eat on the way.

'6–7.30am – I drink three or four cups of coffee during the show. After this I will not have tea or coffee during the day – just water.

'8am – On my way home again and I do not feel like eating.

'10am – I eat something disgusting! Today cold boiled potatoes and the gravy from Sunday's roast! I try to eat one egg a week, but do not eat much bread, which I know is not very good. I do not usually have lunch, but once a week I will have a slap-up meal and not eat in the evening.

'2pm – Usually have some soup. If I am on holiday and feel I need to lose a few pounds I will eat soup for a week.

'4pm – I do not eat any food after this time because I need to be in bed by 9pm, in order to get up at 4am. I work on the theory that my body is parked in the garage while I am in bed so there is no point filling the tank with petrol!

'6pm – I do not answer the telephone after this point in the day; it is now my "quiet time".

'9pm – In bed!

'At weekends I eat pretty normally, with a snack for lunch and proper meal in the evening. I feel my body is just getting back to normal when it is Monday and it goes out of kilter again!'

SARAH KENNEDY has a great start to the day with fruit (a good source of energy and vitamins). She's right to balance her high intake of caffeine during the show by avoiding it for the rest of the day. Soup is also a good idea, as it retains all the nutrients that are lost when we boil vegetables and pour away the cooking water.

★ ★ ★ ★ ★ ★ ★ ★ ★ ★ ★ ★ ★ ★   SARAH KENNEDY

Presenter of BBC Radio 2's *Sarah Kennedy with the Dawn Patrol*

Vegetables and fruit

Write in your total number of portions per day (see page 26) and compare it with the recommended number.

....

Everyone should aim for at least 5 portions a day.

TIPS Iron from meat, fish and alternative protein foods is absorbed better if vegetables and fruit containing vitamin C are eaten at the same time.

Avoid tea for 30 minutes before or after a meal because it inhibits absorption of iron.

continued...

★ ★

 ## Diets are mumbo-jumbo

'All diets are mumbo-jumbo. I have never dieted. I eat what I please. I do not drink as much as I used to and I play golf as often as possible. Apart from that I do not take any exercise.'

Sixty-three year old **MICHAEL PARKINSON** has certainly taken a few steps in the right direction, by drinking less and playing plenty of golf. He's also wise to avoid rapid weight-loss diets which, as we have seen, cause more problems than they solve ...

★ ★ ★ ★ ★ ★ ★ ★ ★ ★ ★ ★ ★ ★ **MICHAEL PARKINSON**

Presenter of BBC Radio 2's *Parkinson's Sunday Supplement*

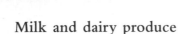

Milk and dairy produce

Write in your total number of portions per day (see page 26) and compare it with the recommended number.

....

Women of all ages, active and sedentary, need about 3 portions per day.

Active men		Sedentary men	
Age	Portions per day	Age	Portions per day
11–14	about 3	11–14	about 3
15–18	about 3	15–18	about 3
19–49	2–3	19–49	2–3

Men of 50+ 2–3 portions per day

- Women, in particular, should eat calcium-rich foods (of which dairy foods are the main source in the UK). Taking in the right amount of calcium, as part of a well-balanced, low-fat diet, along with adequate exercise, will help prevent osteoporosis. Non-dairy sources of calcium include eggs, wholegrain cereals, pulses, nuts, seeds and dark green vegetables.

continued...

Meat, fish and vegetarian alternatives

Write in your total number of portions per day (see page 26) and compare it with the recommended number for your age, sex and level of activity.

....

Active women

Age	Portions per day
11–18	2–3
19–49	2–3

Women of 50+ 2 portions per day

Sedentary women

Age	Portions per day
11–18	2–3
19–49	2

Active men

Age	Portions per day
11–14	3
15–18	4
19–49	2–3

Men of 50 + 2–3 portions per day

Sedentary men

Age	Portions per day
11–14	2–3
15–18	2
19–49	2–3

- Iron is important for preventing anaemia, particularly for women who need more than men, and is most easily and widely available in meat. Vegetarians can obtain iron from pulses and green vegetables.
- Eggs are very nutritious, but do not eat them to the exclusion of other sources of protein (2–4 a week).

continued...

★ ★

★ I'm a nutritional nightmare

'I'm a bit of a nutritional nightmare. I have no breakfast, no lunch and a fairly light dinner of meat and two veg in the evening, which normally means chicken, steak or roast lamb. Either I have found the secret to a healthy, long life or I am a nutritional freak.

'Despite the fact that I broadcast for two hours to the nation, the only thing that keeps me going is the occasional cup of coffee and then only if the famous JY Prog team remember to get me a cup.

'In terms of exercise, I limit this to my short walks between front door and car, and car and studio.

'In spite of this I'm hardly ever ill and have rarely, if ever, missed the JY Prog in 30 years of broadcasting.'

At 73, **JIMMY YOUNG** somehow manages to keep his batteries charged on a regime that would floor most of us. It goes to show that there's always an exception that proves the rule …
At least his one meal is nutritious, though he would probably feel more full of energy and vitality if he added more carbohydrates (potato, pasta, bread) to his main meal and increased his fruit and vegetable intake.

★ ★ ★ ★ ★ ★ ★ ★ ★ ★ ★ ★ ★ ★   JIMMY YOUNG

Presenter of BBC Radio 2's *Jimmy Young* show

Foods containing fats

Write in your total number of portions per day (see page 26) and compare it with the recommended number for your age, sex and level of activity.

....

Active women

Age	Portions per day
11–14	2–3
15–18	2–3
19–49	2–3

Women of 50+ about 1 portion per day

Sedentary women

Age	Portions per day
11–14	1–2
15–18	1–2
19–49	about 1

Active men

Age	Portions per day
11–14	2–3
15–18	4–5
19–49	about 3

Men of 50+ about 1 portion per day

Sedentary men

Age	Portions per day
11–14	about 2
15–18	about 2–3
19–49	1–2

TIP For more information about the type of fats you need see page 62.

continued...

Foods containing sugar

Write in your total number of portions per day (see page 26) and compare it with the recommended number for your age, sex and level of activity.

....

Active women

Age	Portions per day
11–14	1–2 per day
15–18	1–2 per day

Women of 19+ should keep to 0–1 portions to prevent weight gain.

Sedentary women

Age	Portions per day
11–14	0–1
15–18	0–1

Active men

Age	Portions per day
11–14	1–2
15–18	1–2
19–49	1–2

Men of 50+ about 1 portion per day

Sedentary men

Age	Portions per day
11–14	0–1
15–18	0–1
19–49	0–1

TIP It's best to eat sugary foods as part of a meal to reduce the risk of tooth decay.

continued...

Drinks (non-alcoholic)

Write in your total number of drinks per day (see page 26) and compare it with the recommended number.

....

Men and women of all ages should aim to have at least 6–8 drinks, a total of 1.5 litres (2¾ pints) per day, with only up to half being tea or coffee (although you don't have to drink any!). Water is the best drink. Fruit juices and skimmed milk are also good. Limit fizzy and sugary soft drinks.

Alcoholic drinks

Write in your total number of units of alcohol per day (see page 26) and compare it with the recommended number.

....

There isn't really an 'ideal' on this one, and there is no compelling need to take up drinking. If you drink, then 1–3 units per day is fine, but have some alcohol-free days in the week and avoid binges. Benefits to health from alcohol are mainly seen in the over-45s, but women are at more risk from high intake (see page 75).

Putting it together on your plate

Another way of describing a well-balanced diet, in terms of portions of food per day, is to show it as a plate model (see below).

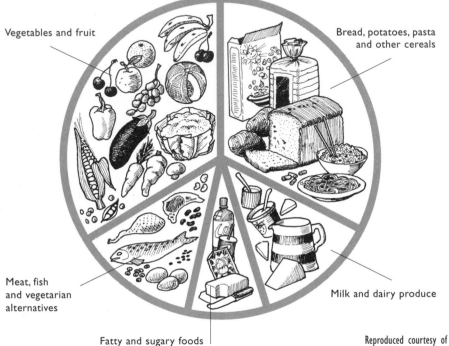

Vegetables and fruit

Bread, potatoes, pasta and other cereals

Meat, fish and vegetarian alternatives

Fatty and sugary foods

Milk and dairy produce

Vegetables and fruit
Choose a wide variety of vegetables and fruit each day.

Bread, potatoes, pasta and other cereals
Starchy foods such as bread, cereals, potatoes, pasta and rice should make up the largest proportion of your food.

Meat, fish and vegetarian alternatives
Eat moderate quantities of lean meat, fish and vegetarian alternatives.

Milk and dairy produce
Eat moderate quantities of low-fat milk and dairy produce and choose lower-fat alternatives whenever you can.

Fatty and sugary foods
You can still enjoy these foods but try not to eat them too often.

Are you the right weight for your height?

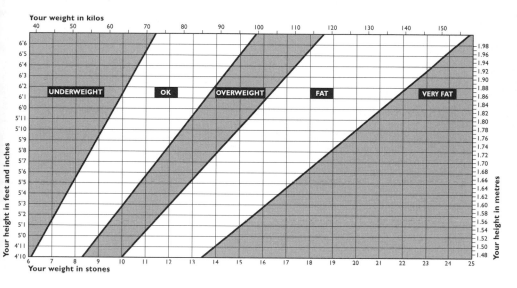

Your weight in kilos

Your weight in stones

Your height in feet and inches

Your height in metres

UNDERWEIGHT　　OK　　OVERWEIGHT　　FAT　　VERY FAT

Reproduced courtesy of the Health Education Authority

We have included this weight chart reluctantly, hoping you will bear in mind the dangers of slavishly following such charts! They can encourage women, in particular, to aim for too low a weight. They also focus teenage girls' attention on their weight at a time when it is desirable for them to deposit a certain amount of fat as their bodies change shape. So, please remember, this chart is really only a guide. It is important not to confuse being at the upper end of your normal weight range, or even being slightly overweight, with being obese.

In fact, there is increasing evidence that being slightly plump might have some health benefits. For example, slightly plump women are less likely to have fertility problems; they give birth to bigger babies (low birth weight is associated with lifelong health problems) and find breast-feeding easier. Plump men and women may also stand a better chance of surviving a heart attack than people who are underweight.

In fact the classic weight and height chart is rapidly going out of fashion, in favour of the Body Mass Index, explained overleaf.

Working out your Body Mass Index

Your Body Mass Index (BMI) gives a good indication of whether you are a healthy weight. To work out your BMI:

1 Work out your height in metres (see the height chart opposite) and multiply the figure by itself.
2 Measure your weight in kilograms.
3 Divide the weight (question 2) by the height squared (i.e. the answer to question 1). For example, you might be 1.6m (5 foot 3 inches) tall and weigh 65kg (10 stone). The calculation would then be: 1.6 x 1.6 = 2.56. Your BMI would be 65 ÷ 2.56 = 25.39.

Now work out your BMI and check your result against the table below. But, before you do, remember not to take it too seriously! Stocky people (and girls, in particular) may appear to be overweight when using this method. So be honest with yourself. If you are naturally of a stocky build do not try to lose weight unnecessarily.

Category	Range
Underweight	Less than 20
Ideal	20–25
Overweight; advisable to lose weight if you are under 50	25–30
You should lose weight	30–40
Definitely too fat; lose weight now	Greater than 40

Height chart

Feet & inches	Metres	Feet & inches	Metres
4' 10"	1.45	5' 9"	1.74
4' 11"	1.5	5' 10"	1.78
5'	1.52	5' 11"	1.8
5' 1"	1.55	6'	1.82
5' 2"	1.57	6' 1"	1.85
5' 3"	1.6	6' 2"	1.88
5' 4"	1.62	6' 3"	1.9
5' 5"	1.65	6' 4"	1.92
5' 6"	1.68	6' 5"	1.95
5' 7"	1.7	6' 6"	1.98
5' 8"	1.72	6' 7"	2

Congratulations, if your BMI is OK. But hang on a minute ...
If your BMI falls within the ideal range and you are the right weight, that's great, but it's still important to eat healthily (see chapter 3) for the vitamins, minerals and other substances needed to keep you fit and well. It is also important not to put on weight. People aged 30 to 74 with BMIs at the lower end of the normal range have the lowest death rates. And people who stay the same weight in middle age as they were in their youth, live longer, are generally healthier and therefore more able to enjoy themselves.

Assessing your waist to hip ratio

As we saw in Chapter 1, your risk of heart disease doesn't only depend on *how much* fat you're carrying – it's also *where* you're carrying it that matters. Our genes determine our basic shape: whether the fat on our bodies is deposited around our hips, breasts and upper arms (women) so that we are pear-shaped; or whether excess fat is deposited on our tummies, making men and some women apple-shaped.

It may seem unfair but if apple-shaped people become overweight they are at greater risk of heart disease and diabetes than pear-shaped people.

To find out which category you fit into:

1 Measure your waist and hips.
2 Then divide the waist measurement by the hip measurement to get your waist–hip ratio.

For example, if your waist is 86cm (34 inches) and your hips 102cm (40 inches), your waist–hip ratio will be 86 ÷ 102 = 0.85. If the ratio of your waist to hip measurement is more than 0.95 as a man and more than 0.87 as a woman you are apple-shaped.

There is another rule of thumb as far as waist measurements are concerned. If a man has a waist that measures more than 94cm (37 inches), or if a woman's is more than 80cm (31 inches), they are categorized by some doctors as overweight. Waists do thicken with age, a phenomenon often referred to as 'middle age spread'. If you are younger and already have a 'spare tyre' – act now! It is this abdominal fat that increases the risk of heart disease.

Where do you go from here?

Having assessed your eating habits and checked your height, weight, waist and hip measurements, you should be able to give an honest answer to the questions:

1 Do I need to lose weight?
2 Do I need to change my eating habits?

Chapter 3

Getting the Measure of Healthy Eating

The average adult in the UK would benefit from:

- Doubling their intake of fruit and vegetables to a minimum of 5 portions a day, making a total of around 400g (14oz)
- Doubling their intake of starchy (carbohydrate) foods to 6–14 portions a day, making a total of 600–800g (1lb 5oz–1lb 12oz)
- Limiting meat and vegetarian alternatives to 3–4 portions a day
- Limiting dairy foods to 2–3 portions a day
- Limiting fats and fatty foods to 1–5 portions a day
- Limiting sugar and foods containing sugar to 0–2 portions a day
- Limiting salt to around 1 teaspoon per day or less

Choosing from a wide variety of foods ensures that you benefit from a wide range of nutrients. It also makes your meals more exciting, colourful and tasty.

Eaten in the right quantities, foods from the four main food groups provide the vitamins, minerals and other components we need for optimum health and vitality, and for looking and feeling great.

Starchy carbohydrate foods — 6—14 portions a day

Starchy foods should make up more than one-third of a healthy diet. This food group includes pasta, bread, rice and other cereals, and also potatoes and other starchy vegetables. They are the best foods for energy. They also contain B vitamins, which help release that energy and are vital for healthy nerves and digestion.

The wide variation in the number of portions of starchy food, between 6 and 14, may seem odd, but is explained by individual needs. For example, a marathon runner using pasta to build an energy store, or a teenager during a growth spurt, might eat 14 portions of starchy foods a day whereas a sedentary woman would need only 5—7 portions per day.

What is a portion of starchy food?

- 3 tablespoons breakfast cereal
- 2 tablespoons muesli
- 1 slice of bread or toast
- 1 bread roll, bap or bun
- 3 crackers or crispbreads

- 1 medium potato
- 2 heaped tablespoons boiled rice
- 3 heaped tablespoons boiled pasta
- 1 medium plantain or sweet potato

Which types of starchy food should you choose?

- Try to eat wholemeal, wholegrain, brown or high-fibre varieties of bread, breakfast cereal, pasta and rice whenever possible. This is because the grains are 'whole' – they have not had the fibre or vitamins and minerals refined out of them. Choose lower-fat sauces for pasta and rice.
- If you do not like wholemeal, try to find another type of high-fibre bread.
- Eat white bread if you do not like brown breads, but try to include some other wholegrain cereals (e.g. breakfast cereals or brown rice or pasta).
- Get into the habit of eating breakfast cereals regularly. Choose ones that are fortified with folic acid (see pages 52–53), other B vitamins and minerals such as iron – these cereals are particularly good for children and for women who may be slimming or whose diets lack iron.

- Porridge is an excellent breakfast cereal because the naturally occurring oatbran is not removed during processing. The gummy fibre lowers blood cholesterol levels, and oats are rich in vitamins and minerals and are a very good source of energy.

Ways to make more of starchy foods

- Make bread, pasta, potatoes or rice the main part of most of your meals. (See Ainsley's recipe for Red Stripe Linguine with Chestnut Mushrooms and Basil, p. 185.)
- Serve larger portions of bread, pasta, rice and potatoes.
- Make more frequent use of noodles and bread made from other wholegrains, such as rice or buckwheat.
- You can eat breakfast cereal at any time of day (as a snack, for instance, to fill up hungry teenagers after school).
- Try using different varieties of rice, e.g. long-grain (brown or white) for pilau; short-grain for paella; brown rice for salads; arborio, carnaroli or other speciality risotto rices; wild rice with fish.
- Try using sweet potato, plantain or yam sometimes, instead of potato. (See Ainsley's recipe for Plantain, Pumpkin and Chickpea Curry, p. 168.)
- Leave the skins on potatoes.

Why is fibre so important?

Fibre in starchy foods is probably best known for preventing constipation but people who eat a high-fibre diet also have a lower risk of heart disease. This is because eating enough fibre reduces our levels of harmful types of blood cholesterol, and it may also help to regulate our blood pressure. By lowering blood cholesterol, fibre may also help prevent gallstones.

To prevent constipation, fibre bulks and softens food waste as it passes through the gut. This can prevent diverticular disease and help control some types of irritable bowel syndrome. Preventing constipation also helps avoid piles and varicose veins.

Fibre protects against colon cancer by encouraging healthy gut bacteria to grow, thereby suppressing harmful gut bacteria (which may be

How much fibre do you need?

The average person needs to eat around 18 grams of fibre per day. The best way is to eat fibre where it occurs naturally – for instance, in starchy foods, vegetables and fruits.

Quick fixes to meet your daily fibre needs:
- 2 Shredded Wheat, a medium portion of wholemeal pasta, an orange and a generous serving of broccoli
- 2 digestive biscuits and a medium portion of baked beans with two slices of wholemeal toast
- 2 Weetabix, a slice of wholemeal toast, a small packet of nuts and a medium portion of brown rice risotto
- A bowl of All-Bran and 3 dried apricots

Good sources of fibre include:
Wholemeal and wholegrain breads, wholemeal pasta, brown rice, pulses (lentils and beans), vegetables, fruit, dried fruit, nuts and seeds, wholemeal flour, soya flour, rye flour, oats and oatmeal, oatcakes, breakfast cereals, millet, barley.

an additional risk factor in heart disease). Eating enough fibre may also help guard against breast cancer, either directly or indirectly. Women who eat more vegetables and fruit and starchy wholegrain cereals have a lower incidence of breast cancer, whereas a high intake of red meat and fried/browned food may increase the risk.

Carbohydrate loading for sport

Athletes are great fans of starchy food. Most elite athletes eat a high-carbohydrate diet for a few days before an endurance event. This is called carbohydrate loading. They also eat a starchy pre-event meal, to boost their energy and endurance. The body turns the starches into glucose and glycogen, to provide both instant and stored energy for the brain and muscles. Starches are a better source of energy than sugar because they contain fibre, vitamins and minerals.

Most of us don't need to eat the massive quantities of carbohydrates consumed by top athletes. But we can all benefit from a bit of carbohydrate loading after exercise, when a starchy snack (as opposed to sugary confectionery or drinks or fatty food) is a better way of replenishing depleted energy. A banana and some water is a lot less expensive than a fashionable sports drink – and does the job of rehydrating and boosting energy very efficiently.

Vegetables and fruit – at least 5 portions a day

Fruit is the ultimate convenience food, requiring little or no preparation. It is easy to carry and enjoyable to eat any time, anywhere, making it a versatile snack. Vegetables are an integral part of all healthy meals. For optimum vitality, five portions of vegetables and fruit per day are recommended – and there is probably even more benefit in eating more, if you want to. Because most fruit can be eaten raw, and many vegetables can be eaten raw in salads or lightly cooked, they retain all their vitamins and minerals, which in other foods are depleted or destroyed by cooking.

Vegetables and fruit include all fresh, frozen, chilled and canned varieties (with the exception of potatoes, which are a starchy food). Also included are dried fruits and fruit juice, but not fruit *drinks* which contain very little, if any, fruit juice and a lot of added sugars or sweeteners and other non-nutritious ingredients.

GETTING THE MEASURE OF HEALTHY EATING

 ## The GI factor

When we eat starchy foods they release energy, in the form of glucose, into the bloodstream, thus raising our blood sugar levels. A slow increase in blood sugar is much healthier than a sudden rise, and this effect is measured by the Glycaemic Index (GI).

Low-GI means a food breaks down slowly during digestion, releasing energy gradually into the bloodstream, resulting in a smaller rise in blood sugar. High-GI means eating a food results in a large and sudden rise in blood sugar. Low-GI foods can help control hunger, appetite and weight and they may help lower raised blood fats and improve sensitivity to insulin (helping to control diabetes and possibly helping to prevent maturity-onset diabetes).

Of all the starchy staples, pasta – both fresh and dried – has the lowest GI score. The GI score of potatoes and rice varies between varieties. But, regardless of GI score, bread, potatoes, pasta and rice are all very valuable foods.

★ ★

★ Three meals a day

'I am a firm believer in three proper meals a day. Breakfast is a hearty affair with fresh orange juice, cereal with semi-skimmed milk and two slices of Granary toast with low-fat spread and camomile tea.

'I used to drink coffee, but following a recent illness I have switched to camomile tea and I feel much better for it.

'For lunch I like a plate of cold meat or fish and a salad.

'Dinner is at 8.30pm and includes lots of vegetables.

'I avoid all fried food – although I do steal the odd chip or two when I'm in the BBC canteen.'

Another member of the BBC Radio 2 broadcasting team, 72 year old **DAVID JACOBS** is a nutritionist's dream! His breakfast menu is particularly good – fresh orange juice for vitamin C, plenty of high-energy, high-fibre carbohydrate in the form of cereal and Granary toast, and low-fat spread and semi-skimmed milk. Eating as healthily as he does, David could even treat himself to his own portion of chips now and then, especially if he does some regular exercise ...

★ ★ ★ ★ ★ ★ ★ ★ ★ ★ ★ ★ ★ ★ | **DAVID JACOBS**

Presenter of BBC Radio 2's *Easy Does It* and
The David Jacobs Collection

What is a portion of fruit and vegetables?

- 1 medium portion of vegetables or salad
- 1 piece of fresh fruit
- 6 tablespoons stewed or canned fruit – 140g (5oz)
- 1 small glass of fruit juice – 100ml (3½fl oz)

How can you eat 5 portions a day and still eat normally?

Here's how five portions a day can fit easily into a normal day's eating:

Breakfast – A glass of fruit juice, or a piece of fruit alone or chopped into cereal.

Lunch – A piece of fruit (after sandwiches etc).

Main meal – Two portions of vegetables (fresh, frozen or canned), in addition to fish, meat or other protein and potatoes.

Pudding – A fruit-based pudding at one meal. (See Ainsley's recipe for Iced Fresh Fruit Platter with Passionfruit Cream, p. 179).

And don't worry – eating five portions a day won't make you overweight because vegetables and fruit are low in calories. If anything, it should help you lose weight because you'll get into the habit of reaching for fruit (instead of sugary, fatty snacks) when you need an energy boost.

Ways to eat more vegetables and fruit

- Eat some raw vegetables and fruit on a daily basis. Seasonal produce is cheaper and tends to be fresher.
- Serve a salad on the side each day with main meals or with light meals such as sandwiches or cheese on toast.
- Serve two portions of vegetables (in addition to potatoes) at every main meal.
- Increase the amount of vegetables and salad ingredients that you include when making sandwiches and packed lunches.
- If you use ready-made salads such as coleslaw, choose the lower-calorie/lower-fat versions or make them go further by adding extra grated carrot. Make your own coleslaw and dress it with natural yoghurt or fromage frais, instead of mayonnaise, to reduce fat.

★ ★

★ Oranges are the only fruit (for breakfast)

'I may have an orange for breakfast and I drink orange juice all through the morning, but I do not usually eat anything until I come off air at 12 noon. I think better on an empty stomach. If I had breakfast I would probably fall asleep!

'For lunch I have a sandwich and then have a meal in the early evening. I do not eat much red meat these days and I try to avoid fried foods, although I do have a weakness for fried bacon.

'My other weakness is snacks – crisps, nuts and occasional pints of beer. If I feel the waistband tightening I spend a week on chicken salad.'

BBC Radio 2 presenter **KEN BRUCE** certainly isn't short of vitamin C! Most people do better with a high-carbohydrate breakfast but 47 year old Ken probably relies on the sugar in the orange juice to keep him going. A sandwich makes a quick, healthy lunch and avoiding fried foods is a good idea – grilled bacon tastes just as good as fried!

★ ★ ★ ★ ★ ★ ★ ★ ★ ★ ★ ★ ★ ★ ★ 　**KEN BRUCE**

Ken Bruce presents the mid-morning slot on BBC Radio 2

- Add lots of vegetables to ready-prepared meals, pasta sauces, pizza toppings, stews, casseroles and even other meat dishes. Family members who 'don't like vegetables' might not be so reluctant to eat them if they are part of a prepared dish. Grated carrot, parsnip and swede, for example, can be incorporated into dishes such as shepherd's pie, lasagne, curries and moussaka.
- Take advantage of the convenience of frozen vegetables which can be cheaper than fresh – and there is no preparation and no waste. Unlike canned vegetables they do not have added salt or sugar. And they contain more vitamins and minerals than tired 'fresh' produce.

- Serve crudités (sticks of carrot, celery, cucumber and other vegetables of your choice, plus radishes) as snacks or in place of crisps and other nibbles.
- If you make your own bread/fruit cake/fruit loaf, add grated carrot.

Why are vegetables and fruit so good for you?

Vegetables and fruit are good for you because they contain vitamins, minerals and other substances that act as antioxidants in your body. Antioxidants help prevent heart disease, cancer and other diseases.

The main antioxidant nutrients are beta-carotene (the pigment that gives orange, yellow and red fruit and vegetables their colour), vitamins C and E and the minerals selenium, zinc, manganese and copper. There are also other substances in fruit and vegetables that act as antioxidants.

Antioxidants are important to health because they neutralize free radicals. Free radicals are highly reactive molecules that are produced naturally when you breathe oxygen and burn food and when the body is under certain kinds of stress such as smoking and pollution. However, if your diet does not provide enough antioxidants to neutralize the amount of free radicals present then they can damage the DNA in cells. This may speed up the ageing process and trigger some cancers. Free radical damage also increases the risk of heart disease by oxidizing cholesterol, making it more likely to be deposited in the arteries.

In addition to the antioxidant role of these nutrients in vegetables and fruit, vitamin C is vital for immunity and healing, and vitamin E (found in some fruit and vegetables but mainly in vegetable oils) strengthens blood capillary walls.

Folates in green vegetables help prevent anaemia and are recommended for pregnant women (see page 53). Folates also have an antioxidant role. Eating unpeeled fruit, and eating the skins of vegetables where appropriate, also provides very palatable dietary fibre. Vegetables and fruit are also a good source of the mineral potassium which may help to lower the risk of stroke by counterbalancing the consumption of too much sodium (see page 70). And some vegetables and fruit are especially rich sources of carbohydrates for energy, particularly bananas, dates and pears.

Super fruit

All fruit is good for you but some fruits contain more nutrients than others. Some can even provide, in one average portion, more than 100 per cent of the Recommended Nutrient Intake (RNI) of particular vitamins. The RNI is the amount of a vitamin or mineral thought to be sufficient each day, even for people with high requirements. Other fruits contribute significant amounts of nutrients. Here are some of the best:

Apples (and citrus fruits) are rich in pectin, the gummy fibre that can help lower blood cholesterol levels.

Apricots (and other dark orange fruit such as peaches and mangoes) are a good source of the antioxidant beta-carotene, the natural plant pigment that gives orange fruit its colour. It is also turned into vitamin A in the body, which is needed by the immune system and for healthy eyes. Apricots also provide a steady stream of energy.

Bananas are full of energy and are a good source of potassium and B vitamins – vital for releasing energy from food during digestion.

Blackcurrants are very high in vitamin C, containing 4½ times the RNI of vitamin C in a 100g (3½oz serving). They also contain good amounts of vitamin E, which is not commonly found in fruit and is protective against heart disease, stroke and cancer.

Dried fruit (such as prunes, pears, apricots, peaches, raisins) is a good source of potassium. Dried apricots are one of the richest fruit sources of iron which is essential to prevent anaemia and symptoms of tiredness, general fatigue and poor immunity.

Oranges and other citrus fruits are an excellent source of vitamin C. Vitamin C boosts the immune system giving protection against infection. It is also needed for strong blood vessels and a glowing skin. As an antioxidant, vitamin C scavenges free radicals (see left) produced as part of normal body chemistry. One medium-to-large orange provides 80mg of vitamin C, twice the RNI. The pith in oranges, and other citrus fruits, is also a source of protective bioflavonoids.

Facts

 ## Are organic fruit and vegetables better for you?

Not eating enough fruit and vegetables is more harmful to health than any hazards from pesticide residues. Government regulations are designed to minimize residues in fruit which, surveillance shows, do not usually exceed Maximum Residue Levels (MRL). However, there are still unanswered questions over long-term exposure to low doses and cocktail effects (the combined effects of several residues).

Thorough washing can remove some of the surface pesticides, fungicides, waxes and other treatments, but cannot remove systemic pesticides (those taken into the plant during growth). If you plan to use the zest or peel of citrus fruit it is wise to use organic or unwaxed fruit, as the waxes contain fungicide. Government advice is to peel and top and tail carrots when feeding babies because of continuing problems with pesticide residues. Parents may also want to peel other non-organic fruit and vegetables for young children.

Comparisons show that organic produce (grown without chemical pesticides and inorganic fertilizers) contains more vitamins and minerals.

Why does folic acid help prevent heart disease?

Ask most people what puts them at greatest risk of a heart attack and they will probably say 'cholesterol'. There are many other risk factors (such as smoking, high blood pressure, obesity, high salt intake and high (saturated) fat intake), but it is cholesterol that has become synonymous with heart attacks.

Yet a raised level of homocysteine seems to be more closely associated with increased risk of heart disease, and particularly stroke, than raised blood cholesterol levels.

Homocysteine is an amino acid, a building block of protein. Like cholesterol, it is essential for normal body function, but having too much causes problems. Raised levels seem to occur when the diet does not provide enough folic acid and, less importantly, two other B vitamins (B6 and B12), to clear the system of homocysteine.

Unlike raised blood cholesterol levels, which are quite hard to reduce through weight loss, diet and exercise, homocysteine levels can be lowered quickly and easily by taking an extra 200 micrograms (mcg) of folic acid a day, in addition to the RNI which is also 200mcg per day for everyone aged eleven years and over (except pregnant and pre-conceptual women, see below).

Scientists estimate that up to half the population has raised levels of homocysteine. So, should we all be taking folic acid supplements? Probably not, because studies have shown that eating just two 30g servings a day of breakfast cereal fortified with folic acid increases intake enough to bring blood levels up to beneficial levels within eight weeks.

Foods fortified with folic acid are marked with a large blue 'f' symbol. Foods labelled 'contains extra folic acid' contain 100mcg of folic acid per portion and those labelled 'contains folic acid' contain 33mcg per portion. These foods are mainly breads and breakfast cereals. In the USA all flour has to be fortified with folic acid by law.

Why do women need folic acid in pregnancy?

Women who are planning a pregnancy are advised to take folic acid tablets from before conception (as soon as you start trying) to the twelfth week of pregnancy, to reduce the risk of spina bifida and related conditions.

The central nervous system is one of the first to develop in the foetus – hence the need for folic acid supplements before and early in pregnancy.

Super veg

Parents have told children for generations that they should eat up their greens if they want to be 'big and strong', so the idea of super veg is nothing new. What is new, is that nutritionists have identified around 500 phyto (plant) chemicals and are beginning to understand their roles. So it is now possible to explain exactly why we should eat up our greens ...

Broccoli and family contain sulphur compounds which seem to protect against cancer, particularly colon cancer (in addition to protection from their fibre content). Cabbage, cauliflower, Brussels sprouts and kale are also good sources of folates, the plant form of folic acid (see opposite). In addition, green leafy vegetables contain a lot of chlorophyll, the pigment that allows green plants to make energy from sunlight, which may help protect against the DNA damage that can lead to cancer.

Garlic, onions, shallots, leeks, spring onions and chives also contain sulphur compounds that may increase cancer resistance. In addition, they have been shown to help lower blood cholesterol levels and blood pressure – although this is a controversial area.

Pumpkin, squash and dark yellow or orange sweet potatoes are good sources of the antioxidant beta-carotene.

Red and green peppers are rich in vitamin C and beta-carotene.

Tomatoes get their colour from lycopene, which is a powerful antioxidant. Cooking and processing tomatoes releases lycopene from their skin so there are higher levels in pasta sauce, tomato ketchup, canned tomatoes, passata and tomato soup than in raw tomatoes. American studies (sponsored by Heinz) have shown that men with higher blood levels of lycopene have half the risk of heart disease. Men who eat tomato products more than twice a week are also at less risk of prostate cancer than men who never eat them.

Obviously for any food to have an effect on health it needs to be eaten regularly and in quantity. See page 142 for methods of preparing and cooking vegetables that help retain their nutrient content.

Facts

Do vitamin pills work in place of fruit and veg?

Taking vitamin and mineral supplements may seem like a short cut to benefiting from the nutrients in fruit, vegetables and other foods. But vitamins and minerals work in combination with fibre and other substances that occur naturally in plants, to boost vitality and give protection. It is probably the combination of all these factors that reduces the risk of cancer and heart disease among people who eat a lot of starchy foods and fruit and vegetables. Purified and synthetic vitamins and minerals in tablet form cannot offer this advantage.

Without daily folic acid tablets of 400mcg or 0.4mg daily, which cost around 4p a day (depending on brand), every baby is potentially at risk.

In addition to taking supplements, you should also eat plenty of foods rich in folates. (There is no danger of overdosing by eating more.)

The following foods contain 50–100mcg per average serving, with the highest listed first: cooked black-eyed beans, Brussels sprouts, beef and yeast extracts, cooked kidney, kale, spinach, spring greens, broccoli and green beans.

The following foods have less folic acid but are still useful sources, containing 15–50mcg per serving: cooked soya beans, cauliflower, cooked chick peas, potatoes, iceberg lettuce, oranges, peas, orange juice, parsnips, baked beans, wholemeal bread, cabbage, yoghurt, white bread, eggs, brown rice and wholegrain pasta.

Many breads and breakfast cereals are fortified with folic acid.

Warning: Liver is a rich source of folates but it should not be eaten by pre-conceptual or pregnant women because it contains between 12 and 20 times the recommended daily allowance of vitamin A. Too much vitamin A can cause serious birth defects.

There is no danger of going short of vitamin A in a well-balanced diet because the body can turn beta-carotene (found in orange and green fruit and vegetables) into vitamin A if it is needed. Pre-conceptual and pregnant women should also avoid liver pâté and sausage. But liver and liver products are safe for non-pregnant breast-feeding women.

Dairy foods – 2–3 portions of lower-fat versions a day

Milk, cheese, yoghurt and fromage frais are all good sources of calcium for strong bones and teeth. And it's not just children who need calcium. Because bones and teeth are living, people of all ages have constant calcium needs. Dairy foods also provide protein for growth and repair, and vitamins A and D for eyes and teeth. While everyone over the age of five would benefit from lower-fat versions, infants and children up to the age of two need full-fat versions.

What is a portion of dairy foods?
- 1 medium glass of milk – 200ml (⅓ pint)
- 1 matchbox-sized piece of Cheddar-type cheese – 40g (1½oz)
- 1 small pot of yoghurt, cottage cheese or fromage frais – 125g (4½oz)

Why are lower-fat dairy foods better for you?
Dairy foods do not contribute as much fat to most diets as meat, but over time swapping to low-fat milk, yoghurt, cheese, fromage frais and desserts will reduce fat in your diet, especially saturated fat. Too much fat (and saturated fats in particular) increases the risk of heart disease and some cancers. Too much fat also contributes to excess weight and all its associated health problems. (For more on the different varieties of fat, see page 64.)

Which milk should you choose?

- Full-fat milk contains 22g fat per pint.
- Semi-skimmed milk contains 9g fat per pint.
- Skimmed milk contains 0.6g fat per pint.

If you have always used whole milk, semi-skimmed does not take much adjusting to because it tastes almost the same. Skimmed milk has a much thinner taste and it takes longer to get used to it. Both contain as much calcium and protein as whole milk. If you really cannot get used to the taste of skimmed milk for use throughout the day, you could use it in cooking and drinks where you won't notice the difference in flavour. But remember that children need full-fat milk until they are two years old.

Meat, fish and vegetarian alternatives — 2–4 portions a day

Many of us enjoy eating meat, although not always in the right proportion to other foods. A quick glance back to the plate model (see page 36) shows the healthy balance of meat on your plate is less than many people think. While meat is nutritious, meat products contain a lot of fat — especially saturated fat. Healthy eating involves moderating the amount (and type) of fat we eat. In general, we need to cut down from our current total of 40 per cent of our calories coming from fat to 35, or even 30, per cent. Meat-eaters get a hefty whack of their fat intake from meat products, which provide 25 per cent of the fat in the typical UK diet.

★ ★

★ Savoury tastes, but no meat or salad

'I do not eat meat. I think it's something to do with being born at the end of the war when meat was rationed. The first time I saw a butcher's shop I thought it was a mistake!

'I am fortunately not into chocolate and sweets. And I do not snack between meals or eat desserts. However, give me some crisps or dips or cheese and I will devour the lot in record time!

'For breakfast I have toast with hummus and a cup of tea. After that I drink coffee throughout the day. I'm proud to be a caffeine addict. I do not believe in drinking 2 litres of water a day – it's a bit of a con as far as I am concerned.

'For lunch I have something light; soup and cheese in winter or fruit in summer, while I do the Daily Mail *crossword. For dinner I eat out a lot – far too much to be healthy. If it's after the show I can be eating dinner as late as 11.30 or midnight. I enjoy all the sauces with whatever the meal is and I love curries.*

'I don't believe in salads either – they are unbelievably tasteless and unappetizing!'

BBC Radio 2 presenter **DON MACLEAN** sounds as if he doesn't have much time for this 'healthy eating lark' but his diet is healthier than he thinks. Toast and hummus is an excellent breakfast – high in carbohydrate, protein and fibre. A warming soup for lunch in winter, and fruit in summer, also sound good. As for curries and sauces, there's no reason why healthy food shouldn't be tasty food, as long as it's not too high in fat. The only worries are Don's very high caffeine intake and his intense hatred of salads. Yet Ainsley's recipes (see page 152) show just how mouthwatering those plates of 'rabbit food' can be!

★ ★ ★ ★ ★ ★ ★ ★ ★ ★ ★ ★ ★ ★

DON MACLEAN

Presenter of BBC Radio 2's *Good Morning Sunday*

What is a portion of meat or protein alternatives?

- 3 medium slices beef, pork, ham, lamb, liver, kidney, chicken or oily fish – 50–70g (2–3oz)
- 115–150g (4–5oz) white fish (not fried in batter)
- 3 fish fingers
- 2 eggs (up to 4 a week)
- 5 tablespoons baked beans or other cooked pulses, lentils, dhal – 200g (7oz)
- 2 tablespoons nuts, peanut butter or other nut products – 60g (2¼oz)

Eat meat, not meat products

If you enjoy meat, the best type to eat is lean meat and not fatty meat products which short-change you on the amount of meat they contain. Meat products include sausages, pâté, meat pies, meat pastes, burgers, koftas, keemas, black and white pudding, faggots, frankfurters, haggis, luncheon meat, meat paste, polony, salami, saveloy and so on …

Why are meat and protein alternatives good for you?

We need to eat moderate amounts of lean meat, fish and vegetarian alternatives because they are good sources of protein which we need for growth and repair. Meat also provides iron and vitamin B12 which prevent anaemia, plus zinc. Magnesium is another mineral found in meat, which works with other ones to promote growth, healthy bones and skin.

How much meat should you eat?

Healthy eating guidelines suggest that if you eat an average amount of meat – 8–10 portions a week or 90g (3oz) a day of red meat (such as beef, lamb, pork or veal), you should not eat any more. If you eat 12–14 portions a week you should cut down in order to reduce your risk of colon cancer, and possibly of breast, prostate and pancreatic cancer. Meat-eaters should also eat lots of vegetables, fruit and starchy foods. Two portions of protein food per day is thought to be enough for most people, but if you are very active you might need more.

Is organic meat any healthier?

Free-range and organic meat should contain less saturated fat and more unsaturated fats than intensively reared livestock that is unable to exercise. Physical activity benefits the health of the animals and also the health of people who eat their meat. However, some of the older/rarer breeds favoured by organic and free-range meat producers are less lean than breeds used in intensive farming.

Organic meat should certainly be free from veterinary drug residues. These are monitored and controlled by government surveillance systems (in the same way that pesticide and other agrochemical residues in fruit and vegetables are). But there are concerns that antibiotic residues in particular may cause resistance problems among people who eat meat. Organic livestock are not routinely given veterinary drugs. Organic farmers also maintain that any link between red meat and cancer is more likely to be due to drug/hormone residues rather than the red meat itself.

The advice to limit or reduce meat consumption, and the link between meat and cancer risk, has (not surprisingly) been challenged by the meat industry whose experts counter that there is no need to reduce meat intake if adequate vegetables and fruit are being consumed to offset any effect from a higher intake of meat.

Swap meat for fish

Fish is an excellent low-fat protein food. White fish (e.g. cod, haddock and plaice) is especially low in fat and rich in minerals including iodine. Oily fish (such as mackerel, salmon, tuna, sardines and herring) has the advantage of being rich in essential polyunsaturates called omega-3 fatty acids. These are different from the polyunsaturates found in vegetable oils, but do not worry if you are a vegetarian or cannot eat fish, because the fatty acids contained in green leafy vegetables, vegetable oils and margarine can be used in a similar way by your body (provided you eat a well-balanced diet that is not too high in saturated/trans fats, see page 64).

Omega-3 oils make the blood less sticky and therefore less likely to clot and cause a heart attack. They also help reduce blood pressure. A proportion of omega-3 oils survive canning so canned oily fish (like tuna, pilchards, sardines and herring) will still benefit your health.

In addition, oily fish contain the fat-soluble vitamins A and D. And canned fish (e.g. sardines and pilchards) are rich in calcium, phosphorus and fluoride because the bones are edible.

To benefit from fish, it needs to be a regular part of your diet. Replacing two meat meals a week with fish, making one of them oily fish, is a good way to start. It also replaces the saturated fat in meat with unsaturated fat and lowers your overall fat intake.

Full of beans

Replacing some meat or meat products, or extending meat dishes with pulses, nuts or seeds, are also good ideas. Vegetarians, in particular, should eat at least 30g (1oz) pulses per day. Pulses are fantastically versatile, low in fat, high in protein and fibre. Yet most people don't eat enough of them. Combined with cereal products (like bread or pasta) and grains (rice, couscous, etc), beans provide amino acids (the building blocks of protein) in the right proportions to make them an excellent vegetarian protein alternative to meat. Beans also provide B vitamins for healthy nerves and digestion, fibre and minerals such as iron to help prevent anaemia. And soy protein has other health benefits too.

Ways of using more beans and pulses

- Baked beans are a good convenience food and they can be put in sauces and casseroles.
- Take advantage of other canned pulses (such as red kidney, cannellini and flageolet beans) because starting from scratch involves long cooking times, especially for chickpeas and soy beans.
- Pulses can form the basis of soups (such as minestrone), stews and casseroles.
- Cooked beans and lentils make very tasty salads – add celery, carrot, parsley, sweetcorn and spring onions, and bind with a fromage frais or yoghurt dressing, or a low-fat vinaigrette. (See Ainsley's recipe for Cor! Puy Lentil, Red Onion and Sun-dried Tomato Salad, p. 159.)
- Ethnic dishes offer exciting ways to enjoy pulses. For example, you could try dhal and other lentil and pulse curries, Mexican tacos and refried beans, and Chinese or Japanese recipes that use tofu (bean curd) and tempeh (both made from soy beans). (See Ainsley's recipe for Peppy's Jamaican Rice and Peas, p. 155.)

Foods containing fat – 1–5 portions per day

Although we tend to think that fat is always bad for our health (particularly when it comes to heart disease), the fact is that we *need* fat for its essential fatty acids, fat-soluble vitamins and, for the very young, concentrated calories. It also makes food taste good and has a pleasant 'mouth-feel'. However, most of us would benefit from eating less fat and making sure that most of the fat we do eat is of the unsaturated variety found in vegetable oils.

We need only a small amount of unsaturated fat each day, around 30g (1oz), to enable us to absorb fat-soluble vitamins, but we can 'safely' eat more than that. The maximum amount of fat you need depends on your age, size and how active you are. But, for most sedentary adults to maintain a healthy weight women should eat no more than 70g fat a day, and men 90g.

How can vegetarians get equal nutrients?

Iron in meat and fish is more easily used by the body. The same is true of zinc, another important mineral found in meat. Vegetarian sources of iron include wholegrains, pulses, dried apricots and dark green vegetables. Eating or drinking foods and drinks rich in vitamin C (e.g. orange juice) at the same meal will help improve uptake of vegetarian iron. And avoiding tea or coffee 30 minutes before and after a meal will also help, as these drinks inhibit the absorption of iron.

What is a portion of fats?
- 1 teaspoon margarine or butter
- 2 teaspoons low-fat spread
- 1 teaspoon cooking oil, fat or ghee

What is a portion of fatty foods?
- 1 tablespoon vinaigrette (salad dressing) or mayonnaise
- 1 tablespoon cream
- 1 packet of crisps or other savoury snack
  Other fatty foods include pastry, meat products, sausages, pâtés, fried foods and fatty bacon.

Why should you limit fats in a balanced diet?
Too much fat, and saturated fat in particular, increases the risk of heart disease by raising the level of harmful blood cholesterol. Cholesterol can build up in the arteries, slowing down the blood supply to the heart – or even cutting it off completely, causing a heart attack. Diets high in fat also increase the risk of some cancers.

Not all fats have the same effect. Saturated fats (from animal fats and hydrogenated vegetable fats) cause the most problems. Polyunsaturates (mainly from vegetable oils, except palm and coconut) are essential for health, and can help lower cholesterol levels. Monounsaturates (mainly from olive oil) seem to share the benefits of polyunsaturates. But all fats should be eaten in moderation.

Saturated fats

These are the ones we should be cutting down on. They are mainly found in animal foods such as meat and dairy produce, and they are solid at room temperature (e.g. butter, lard and creamed coconut). Other sources are 'hydrogenated vegetable fats and oils' which are mainly found in hard and some soft margarines, cooking fats, cakes, biscuits, savoury snacks, chocolate and other processed foods and some vegetable oils. These fats are also solid at room temperature.

Monounsaturated fats

These mainly occur in olive oil, groundnut and rapeseed oils, avocados, most nuts and some spreads. They seem to help lower levels of harmful blood cholesterol while not affecting beneficial types of cholesterol, an advantage over too much polyunsaturates. Foods high in monounsaturates also tend to be rich in vitamin E, a nutrient often lacking in the British diet.

Our bodies can make saturated and monounsaturated fatty acids from starchy foods and protein so we do not have to eat them.

Polyunsaturated fats

These are the fats we need to include in our diet because our bodies cannot make some of them. These are called the essential fatty acids. There are two types: omega-6, from vegetable oils such as sunflower; and omega-3, from soya and rapeseed oil, walnuts and oily fish such as mackerel, herring, sardines and salmon. The risk of a heart attack is reduced by these fatty acids, which decrease the tendency of the blood to clot, and their anti-inflammatory action also helps protect against arthritis.

! How many calories are in fat?

Fat contains twice as many calories as starchy foods or protein. Eating less helps you control your weight and improves your health.

Fat = 9 calories per gram

Carbohydrates = 3.75 calories per gram

Protein = 4 calories per gram

Alcohol = 7 calories per gram

Trans fats

These are produced when vegetable oils are hydrogenated (hardened) to make margarine and shortening. They raise levels of the harmful type of cholesterol in our blood, thus increasing the risk of heart disease. They also block production of some essential fatty acids which are particularly important during pregnancy for the healthy development of the baby.

Why is eating less butter and margarine good for you?

Butter, margarine and spreads contribute even more fat to most people's diet than oils (21 per cent from butter and margarine, compared with 14 per cent from cooking oils and fats). If you want to cut down on fat – and saturated fats in particular – it's well worth looking at your intake of this group of foods.

Some people find reduced-fat or low-fat spreads helpful, but they may not be as low in fat as you think. Some terms used on packs, such as 'lite' or 'light', have no legal definition. So, whichever spread you choose – and foods can be very palatable without them – use it sparingly.

The fat content of spreads and oils

The following is an approximate guide to the fat content of the various types of spreads available. However it does not tell you what proportion of the fat in the spread is saturated, unsaturated, monounsaturated or trans fat. That information should be on the label – although not all manufacturers 'own up' on the label to how much trans fat is in their products.

Product	Percentage of fat
Vegetable oils	100
Lard	100
Suet	85
Butter and margarine	80
Spreads	70
Reduced-fat spreads	60
Half-fat spreads	40
Low-fat ('light' 'lite' and 'diet') spreads	40
Very low-fat spreads	25
Extra low, very low-fat spreads	22
Tesco Lowest Ever Fat Spread	5

Easy ways to cut down on fats

Here are some really useful tips for cutting down on the fat in your diet, and for altering the type of fat you use. They may seem like small steps but over time they can make massive savings on the amount of fat you eat and thus reduce your weight and improve your health.

- Cut out the use of lard and other hard fats, as far as possible. Use vegetable oils instead – or soft vegetable-based fats or oils – in cakes and for baking.
- Use a fat replacer for some baking, e.g. Lighter Bake prune purée (sold in supermarkets) replaces some of the fat and sugar in conventional recipes.
- Get into the habit of eating bread without any spread, or dip it in a little olive oil, if you are not trying to lose weight. Bread without a spread is great with soup, with cheese, with cold meat, with hummus and other vegetable spreads and fish pâtés. Breads with some texture and flavour – such as French sticks, Granary loaves, rolls and other speciality breads – taste better this way than sliced bread.
- Try toast without spread when it is topped with moist foods such as baked beans, sardines in tomato sauce or scrambled egg.
- There is no need to automatically butter bread when making sandwiches. Bread is buttered to prevent it soaking up moisture from fillings – making sandwiches nearer to the time they are to be eaten solves this problem. Making them in the morning for lunchtime will be fine – unlike shop-bought sandwiches which are often made three days before you buy and eat them! Butter is also used to make the bread seem less dry. Adding lots of salad filling and grated vegetables gets round this and makes the fillings healthier.
- Vegetables don't need to be covered in butter to taste good. Cook them with spices and herbs for flavour. If you want them to glisten for presentation purposes, brush on a little olive oil, or olive oil mixed with lemon juice – it's lighter, tastier and goes further for fewer calories.

Foods containing sugar – 0–2 portions per day

On average, men eat about 115g (4oz) sugar a day and women eat about 90g (3¼oz) which accounts for around 20 per cent of total calorie intake. Ideally, we should halve our intake to make room for more nutritious, and possibly lower-calorie, foods.

Most of us think of sugar as white or brown sugar, but 'sugar' also includes honey, treacle, syrup, molasses, dextrose, glucose, fructose, maltose, corn syrups, glucose syrups and other industrial sugars added to processed foods.

What is a portion of sugar or sugary foods?

- 1 tablespoon sugar
- 1 rounded teaspoon jam/honey
- 2 biscuits
- 1 slice of cake, or a doughnut or Danish pastry
- 1 small bar of chocolate
- 1 small tube or bag of sweets

Sugar, not so sweet

Although sugar is a carbohydrate, and we should be eating more carbohydrates, sugar is a *refined* carbohydrate. Unlike starchy carbohydrates (see page 42), sugar contains only 'empty' calories – with no vitamins, minerals or fibre to contribute to our health. However, sugar makes many foods taste nicer, and most of us enjoy some sugary food, even if we do not put sugar in tea or coffee. So we're not about to tell you to give up sugar altogether, which some extreme diets recommend.

In fact, slimming plans that contain small quantities of sweet foods have been shown to be more successful than no-sugar or very low-sugar diets because they are easier to stick to. Sweet foods also switch off our appetites more quickly and effectively than fatty foods which are easier to over-eat. So, there is no need to feel guilty about eating some sweet foods as part of a well-balanced diet – just try to avoid frequent sugary snacks between meals, especially because sugar is more likely to give you holes in your teeth than the sugars that occur naturally in fruit, milk or whole starchy foods.

Why is eating less sugar better for you?

Habitually grazing on sugary foods can lead to a dietary vicious circle. Cravings for sweet foods are caused by low blood sugar levels. These are satisfied by eating sugary foods which give a rapid rise in blood sugar, followed by a slump that is lower than the original low that caused the craving.

So, while it is not necessary to regard sugar as 'pure, white and deadly', you should bear in mind that it leaves less room in your diet for more nutritious foods.

Tips for cutting down on sugar

The wonderful thing about our tastebuds is that they are very responsive to change, making it possible to gradually adjust the amount of sugar we use. When the adjustment has been made, what was once 'normal' will taste unpleasantly sweet. Do not try to give up sugar overnight. If you do it gradually you will notice the difference less. And if you have a family, and they are changing their eating habits too, they will be more receptive to gradual change. They might not even notice if you do not mention it. (This is a much better way of doing it than using artificial sweeteners which don't change your underlying tastes and habits.)

- If you sprinkle sugar on to breakfast cereal, gradually cut down on the amount you add until you no longer add any. If you take sugar in tea and coffee, gradually cut down in the same way so that you get used to drinks without sugar. Some people find they can do without sugar in tea more easily than in coffee.
- If you cook with sugar, gradually reduce the quantity. You should eventually be able to eat most cooked fruits (except perhaps rhubarb and gooseberries!) without added sugar.

- Cook fruit in fruit juice or half-juice/half-water rather than sugar syrups.
- Dried fruit can be a useful sweetener. When cooking fruit, for example, you can add raisins to rhubarb or mix chopped dried pears with gooseberries.
- Some spices are also naturally sweet. For example, cinnamon, mixed spice, allspice and ginger can help flavour and 'sweeten' fruit if need be.
- Buy fruits canned in juice rather than syrup.
- Choose unsweetened fruit juice rather than 'fruit juice drinks' which are often sold alongside fruit juice – even in the chiller cabinet – to fool us into buying these over-priced and nutrient-depleted drinks.
- And, given the choice, select sugar-free soft drinks and slimline mixers.

Salt – reduce from 9g per day to around 6g

At the moment we eat about 13g (½oz) of salt a day, which is equivalent to 2½ teaspoons. Around 1 teaspoon a day would be an improvement because all the sodium we need is supplied naturally in the foods that make up the average well-balanced diet.

Is salt the same as sodium?

Confusingly, nutrition panels on food labels give only sodium content. Salt is actually sodium chloride. Sodium, as a mineral, is essential for a variety of body functions. But eating too much, in combination with a low potassium intake and being overweight, can lead to high blood pressure in older people. High blood pressure increases the risk of strokes and heart disease – so it's important to cut down on salt.

Some foods claim to be 'reduced salt' or 'low salt', but this is pretty meaningless when the nutrition panel only lists the sodium content. As a consumer, you might think this is a plot to keep you ignorant of the true amount of salt you are eating. Amazingly enough, it is actually illegal to give the amount of salt in a particular food on the nutrition panel!

Whatever the motives of the government and the food industry, you can work out how much salt is in your food by a simple sum (the salt

Facts

How much salt and sodium should you eat?

Daily salt
Men – less than 7g per day
Women – less than 5g per day

Daily sodium
Men – less than 2.5g per day
Women – less than 2g per day

content equals the sodium content multiplied by 2.5). Or you can memorize the amount of sodium or salt (shown in the box above) that it is advisable to eat per day.

Salt substitutes

Most salt substitutes mix ordinary salt (i.e. sodium chloride) with potassium chloride and/or magnesium sulphate (and other ingredients, such as anti-caking agents), so do not be fooled into thinking you are avoiding salt altogether.

The products vary widely in the amount of sodium they contain. Reduced sodium 'salts' can contain 50 per cent salt, but very low sodium products may contain only 0.9g per 100g sodium, compared with 38.9g in ordinary salt. Some people detect an aftertaste with potassium products in particular.

The sodium/potassium balancing act

Food processing removes the potassium found naturally in foods. Our bodies need potassium to keep sodium in balance. And the best sources of potassium are vegetables, fruit, fish and lean meat.

These fresh foods also leave less room for salty, processed foods in your diet. (As much as *80 per cent* of our salt intake comes from processed foods.)

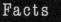

Facts

How much salt is in common foods?

High-salt foods

table/cooking salt

cured/smoked meat

smoked fish

canned meat

cottage cheese

salted butter/margarine/
    spreads

savoury crackers/crisps

salted nuts/savoury
    snacks

some sweet biscuits

baked beans

canned vegetables

olives

sauces (e.g. ketchup,
    Worcestershire sauce,
    brown sauce, soya
    sauce)

stock cubes (unless
    salt-free)

**Moderate to
low-salt foods**

fresh fruit and vegetables

wholemeal flour and pasta

brown rice

breakfast cereals without
    added salt (e.g. puffed
    wheat, Shredded Wheat,
    porridge oats)

unsalted butter and
    low-salt spreads

nuts

dried fruit

pulses

oatmeal and oats

milk

fresh fish

poultry

game

meat

eggs

How you can control your salt intake

Tastebuds respond rapidly to salt – the more you have, the more you want. Gradually cutting down results in what you once found tasty becoming unpleasantly salty. It sounds simple, but if you cut down gradually you can take the whole family with you and avoid alienating everyone.

- Replace canned, pre-packaged, convenience, takeaway and ready-made meals with freshly cooked meals made from fresh/frozen vegetables, fish, poultry and meat.
- Eat more fruit, vegetables and low-salt starchy foods such as rice, pasta, potatoes and bread as part of a balanced diet.
- Gradually cut down on the salt you add during cooking and at the table.

Salty exceptions

The following foods are relatively high in salt but they should not be avoided (unless on doctor's orders), as they provide other important and protective nutrients:

- Bread
- Many breakfast cereals (especially cornflakes)
- Hard cheese
- Some oily fish (e.g. kippers, smoked mackerel and canned fish, especially in brine)

Despite its salt content, which varies widely, bread (for example, in the form of sandwiches) is better than sausage rolls or pie and chips for lunch. And sandwiches or toast are better snacks for children than crisps or confectionery. Breakfast cereal with milk is a very nutritious food for all ages – especially for teenagers who often have erratic eating habits!

Alcoholic drinks – 1–3 per day, with some drink-free days

Moderate drinking, which means 2–3 units per day for women and 3–4 units per day for men (but not necessarily every day), has been associated with reduced risk of heart disease and stroke among men and women over 45.

★ ★

★ # Wine and a salad a day

'I'm not a snacker and I do not eat between meals. For the last 10 years my wife Linda and I have used fresh food and we try to have a salad a day. I also enjoy a glass of wine with lunch and one with dinner. I prefer a larger lunch to dinner as my show is on air at 10.30pm. When I get home after the show I am still buzzing so I potter around and usually have some cheese. I get to bed at 2am and am woken by the children at 6.30am, although I do not get up until 8.30.

'For breakfast once or twice a week I will have scrambled egg (two eggs) but usually cereal, fruit and orange juice. For lunch I have a sandwich with cottage cheese, avocado, mushrooms and tomatoes or pasta – and a glass of wine! Dinner is usually light: fish and potatoes or pasta with a salad or vegetables – and a glass of wine.

'We tried food combining for a while but came to the conclusion that where food is concerned everything in moderation is the best bet.'

Thirty-nine year old **RICHARD ALLINSON** and his family sound as if they enjoy a healthy, varied and delicious diet containing plenty of cereal, bread, pasta, potatoes, eggs, fish, plenty of fruit, vegetables and salad, and wine in moderation. Such a healthy diet makes Richard resilient to working late and being woken early by his children.

★ ★ ★ ★ ★ ★ ★ ★ ★ ★ ★ ★ ★ ★

RICHARD ALLINSON

Richard Allinson hosts a regular evening slot on BBC Radio 2

Mediterranean-style drinking

The healthiest way is to enjoy small amounts of alcohol regularly with food – the pattern of drinking associated with the traditional Mediterranean diet.

Although antioxidants in wine may help reduce the risk of heart disease, any type of alcohol can benefit you by increasing beneficial cholesterol in the blood and slightly decreasing harmful cholesterol.

However, because of other risks associated with alcohol, doctors do not recommend taking up drinking. If you do drink, it should be as part of a well-balanced diet because vitamins and minerals are needed to detoxify the alcohol. Having some alcohol-free days and avoiding getting drunk are also conditions of benefiting from a few drinks!

Women face a greater risk

Women are usually advised to avoid alcohol while trying to become pregnant. While not drinking is probably the ideal, you should not be overly worried if you find you are pregnant and you have been drinking 'normally' up to the time of pregnancy. It would be a good idea to stop drinking if there is a suspicion of pregnancy and, once pregnancy is confirmed, until after the fourth month when 1–2 units per week are thought to be harmless.

Unlike men, the optimum level for women in middle and old age may be lower because of their smaller size and because women are at less risk of heart disease than men. Women are also more susceptible to liver damage and breast cancer, which is increased by about 10 per cent for each additional unit drunk on average per day.

Easy ways of changing your drinking habits

- Introduce drink-free days.
- Pace your drinking so that you drink more slowly.
- Control the amount of nibbling you do when you drink. Nuts, crisps and other salty and savoury snacks will make you thirstier – they are designed to do that to increase your drinking!

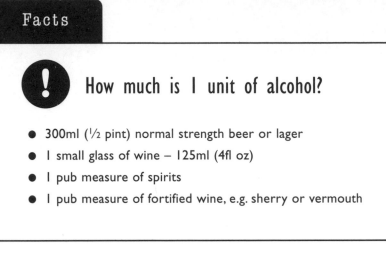

Facts

! How much is 1 unit of alcohol?

- 300ml (½ pint) normal strength beer or lager
- 1 small glass of wine – 125ml (4fl oz)
- 1 pub measure of spirits
- 1 pub measure of fortified wine, e.g. sherry or vermouth

- Eating before you drink will help cut down on nibbles (see previous page) and also ensure that you do not go short of essential vitamins and minerals.
- Eating with alcohol, or before drinking it, is important to slow down absorption.
- Alternate alcoholic drinks with non-alcoholic drinks. (Remember that it takes your body one hour to get rid of 1 unit of alcohol.)
- Make alcoholic drinks last longer by extending them with fizzy mineral water or mixers.

Other drinks

Try to drink at least six to eight cups or mugs or glasses of liquid each day. Not all of them should be tea or coffee because they contain stimulants (such as caffeine) and they are diuretic (make you lose water in urine). Cola and other sweetened fizzy drinks also contain caffeine and sugar or artificial sweeteners and other non-nutritional additives.

Water is the best drink for quenching thirst and hydrating the body. But if you don't like plain water try to replace some of the tea, coffee and colas with other drinks that you like. What about fruit juice or diluted juice? Or try juice drinks or squash or cordials (although these are only around 5 per cent juice and mainly consist of water and sugar or additives). There is also a wide range of herb and fruit 'teas' available which don't contain any caffeine and come in many delicious flavours.

Chapter 4

Do You Need to be More Active? Here's How the Easy Way

The shocking facts about fitness

- Six out of ten men and seven out of ten women in the UK are not active enough to benefit their health.
- Nearly one-third of men and two-thirds of women would find it difficult to walk up a gradual (1:20) slope at a reasonable pace – about 5km (3 miles) per hour. After a few minutes they would need to rest.
- Even walking on level ground at this speed is a severe exertion for many older women, and more than half of women aged 55 to 64 are not fit enough to walk on the level at this speed.
- Because many older people are overweight as well as being unfit, they do not have the muscle strength to do simple tasks like getting out of a chair without using their arms, or climbing the stairs without pulling themselves up, or needing assistance.

You might expect this lack of fitness, shocking though it is, of older people (although older people can be as fit as they were in their twenties). However, many children and younger people, women in particular, are also very unfit. Women aged 16 to 24 are among the least active, whether they are living at home, independent, or with children of their own. But it is not so much lack of exercise as lack of activity that causes these problems. For example, British children do far less physical activity at school than their European classmates – only one-and-a-half hours a week (compared with more than three hours). Children aged eight to 16 spend five times as long watching television as they do being active. And a sedentary childhood can lead to health problems later in life.

★ ★

★ ## I like the buzz of exercise

'I play squash three times a week and that keeps me fit. I really enjoy exercise — I like the buzz after exercise and it is a good idea to keep fit.

'My son is a professional rugby player so we have a lot of gym equipment in the house such as weights and a rowing machine, so I work out on that — in fits and starts.

'As you get older you need to watch your weight because other health problems can occur if you are overweight. Besides, I have a personal horror of getting a big belly! If I want to lose weight I exercise more, I don't believe in diets, although I have a special Chinese diet — eat as much Chinese food as you like, but only use one chopstick!'

If you enjoy the form of exercise you take, you're more likely to stick at it. So it's important to find a sport you genuinely like, especially if you're a busy broadcaster like Don. He gets a real buzz from playing squash and working out on gym equipment at home.

DON MACLEAN
Height: 1.8 metres (5'11½")
Weight: 85kg (13½ stone) *Age:* mid-50s.

★ ★ ★ ★ ★ ★ ★ ★ ★ ★ ★ ★ ★ ★ ★

Fight the Unfitness Epidemic

The fact is, we are experiencing an Unfitness Epidemic. But the good news is that we can improve this by becoming even more moderately active. We do not need to chase tough aerobic targets. Moderate activity can benefit you in so many ways. It can also help you lose weight and maintain weight loss successfully. So, now's the time to become more active.

The Fighting Fat, Fighting Fit Activity Questionnaire

It's easy to dismiss lack of fitness as being other people's problem, but we need to be honest with ourselves. Most of us are not as fit and active as we think we are. Bridging this reality gap is a bit of a challenge. But answering the *Fighting Fat, Fighting Fit* Activity Questionnaire should help.

Contrary to the old maxim 'No Pain, No Gain' (a myth from the seventies when the aerobics craze took off), it definitely does not have to hurt to get fit… and the benefits are tremendous. More activity makes you feel and look good, gives you a sense of achievement and a chance to get out of doors, is fun, relaxing and helps control your weight.

■ How do you rate your level of physical activity?

Circle the letter next to the statement which is closest to how you feel about your level of physical activity:

a I am not currently very physically active, and I do not intend to become more active in the next six months/I'm too busy right now.

b I am not currently very physically active, and I am thinking about increasing the amount of activity I take in the next six months.

c The amount of activity I take varies: sometimes I am physically active, other times not.

d I am currently physically active on most days, but I have only begun to be so within the last six months.

continued…

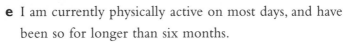

e I am currently physically active on most days, and have been so for longer than six months.

f A year ago I was physically active on most days, but in the last few months have been less active.

2 Consider the last seven days from yesterday. If last week was unusual, for example because you were on holiday, or you couldn't do what you normally do because of illness, think about the last typical week. How many times during the week did you do any of the following vigorous physical activities (activities which made you breathe hard or sweat) for at least 20 minutes continuously:

Running, squash, vigorous swimming, stair-climbing, aerobics, tennis, football, fast cycling, cycling over hilly ground, heavy lifting/carrying, digging.

Circle the number of times per week: 0 1 2 3 4 5 6 7 7+

3 How many times during the week did you do any of the following moderate physical activities (which made you breathe a bit harder, or made you feel warm) for at least 30 minutes (you can count two periods of 15 minutes' continuous activity, as long as they were on the same day):

Brisk walking, easy cycling over flat ground, carrying medium-weight objects, heavy housework (e.g. floor scrubbing), dancing, easy swimming, golf, gentle tennis, cricket.

Circle the number of times per week: 0 1 2 3 4 5 6 7 7+

continued...

How did you score?

If your answer to Question 1 was statement a and you circled 2 or less for Question 2, and 4 or less for Question 3:

As you have probably guessed, you are not active enough at present. Building up to 30 minutes of activity a day will definitely improve your health. You do not need to sweat – the activity only has to be moderate. That means anything which makes you feel warm and makes you breathe slightly more heavily than usual.

Every little bit counts. Even small bouts of activity, spread throughout the day, will help your health in many ways. Being active is fun, it gives you more energy, helps you sleep, helps you relax and gets you out and about to meet friends. Taking more physical activity is a great way to control stress, improve concentration and feel better about yourself. Go on – think about it now. It will add years to your life and life to your years. (For more on the benefits of being active, see page 86.)

If your answer to Question 1 was statement b or statement c and you circled 2 or less for Question 2, and 4 or less for Question 3:

You are probably already thinking about becoming more active and you may even be feeling just about ready to do something about it. But did you realize that probably all you have to do is a little bit more activity, a little more often?

continued...

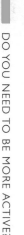

The key to success is to choose activities that you enjoy and that are realistic for you. Why not have a go at building up your everyday activity levels? There are lots of ways to do it.

Why not use the stairs instead of the lift, or walk part or all of the way to work or the shops? Go for a walk at lunchtime – invite a colleague to go with you for a chat on the way. Start slowly and gradually build up the amount you do. You don't have to be a sporty type – any activity is better than none. Nor do you need great chunks of time. Just have fun increasing your activity level in your daily life.

(For more on the benefits of being active, see page 86.)

If your answer to Question 1 was statement d and you circled 3 or more for Question 2 and/or 5 or less for Question 3:

Congratulations. You are already on your way to a healthier active life. Now you have started doing some activity, try to build up to doing 30 minutes of moderate activity on most days of the week. It doesn't matter if progress is slow – any activity is better than none.

Be prepared for setbacks. There will be times when it is difficult to be active – for example, when you go on holiday or when you are particularly busy. Don't worry about it, although you could try to plan ahead. For example, think of what you're going to do on holiday. Could you build in more walks and use the car less? Or, if you are busy at work, could you walk some or all of the way home?

continued...

You could also try setting some goals now which are challenging but realistic and achievable. Keep a record of your activity so you can see your progress. Write down your goals, including the type of activity you want to do and for how long. Keep checking on how well you are achieving these. If they are too difficult, don't give up. Modify your goals to make them slightly easier, before you move on.

You are probably already benefiting from being active by having fun, socializing, feeling less stressed, more energetic, and having better control over your weight.

(For more on the benefits of being active, see page 86.)

If your answer to Question 1 was statement e and you circled 3 or more for Question 2 and/or 5 or less for Question 3:

Well done. You are already leading an active, healthy life. Just keep up the good work!

Here are some tips for the times when it is harder to stay active:

- The main thing is not to worry; recognize these times as temporary setbacks and aim to get back to being active as soon as possible.

- It's a good idea to have a plan 'b' for times when you cannot use your regular form of activity. For example, if you are on holiday or away from work, plan another activity that you can do instead (e.g. swimming, walking or running).

continued...

- Set yourself goals and make them challenging yet achievable, e.g. add extra lengths at the pool.
- Recognize your successes and give yourself small rewards, e.g. a new pair of shorts or shoes.
- Try to build activity into your social life, e.g. active family breaks.
- Remember to be active around the house and office. At work, encourage your employer to put up posters, reminding people to use the stairs rather than the lift.

If your answer to Question 1 was statement f and you circled 2 or less for Question 2 and/or 4 or less for Question 3:

It's a pity that you are no longer as active as you were. But do not worry about it. All sorts of things can interrupt regular activity, such as illness or injury, the demands of home or job, the weather, or the time of year. Try to remember what you liked best about being active. Was it having fun, socializing, the reduction in stress, having more energy or better weight control?

If your circumstances have changed you might want to find a new activity rather than go back to a previous one. Remind yourself that being active is about doing a little more, a little more often. Start again slowly, and gradually build up the amount you do until you are back at the level you were at before, or until you have built up to 30 minutes of moderate activity on at least five days of the week. Try to choose an activity that you enjoy. Good luck.

The facts about exercise

How much exercise and how often?

Experts now agree that 30 minutes of moderate activity at least five days a week significantly improves health and well-being. It can also hold down or prevent weight gain. Combining moderate activity with a calorie-controlled slimming plan certainly helps weight loss.

What is moderate activity?

Moderate activity is any activity that leaves you feeling warm and breathing more heavily than usual. Examples are:

- walking
- golf
- social dancing (e.g. salsa, jive, bhangra, ballroom; line dancing is rather static but would be a good way to start for someone who hasn't exercised before)
- cycling
- table tennis
- aquacise at your local swimming pool
- roller blading (or roller skating)
- heavy DIY (e.g. mixing cement)
- heavy gardening (e.g. digging)
- heavy housework (e.g. spring cleaning)
- sports such as football, swimming, tennis, aerobics and cycling if they are done so that you are not out of breath or sweating profusely
- badminton
- martial arts
- Moderate level alternatives in the *Fighting Fat, Fighting Fit* video. The *Fighting Fat, Fighting Fit* video is a great place to start. It's easy to follow, can be done in parts or as a whole, utilizes objects that you have around you, such as bags and books, to give you strength and demonstrates both vigorous and moderate levels of activity.

How can you build moderate activity into your daily life?

Building moderate activity into your life could involve:

- walking a couple of bus stops
- parking farther from work/shops
- walking instead of sitting in traffic jams
- using the stairs
- washing the car
- doing some gardening or DIY
- spring-cleaning your house
- taking a dog for a walk
- cleaning the windows
- cancelling deliveries and walking to the shops for milk and papers

More than ten good reasons to be more active

1 It will help regulate your appetite, control your weight, and burn fat.

2 Regular exercise develops and tones muscles, giving you a better figure. Muscle also burns more calories than fat, helping you keep in shape.

3 It protects you against a whole host of illnesses, including heart disease, stroke, high blood pressure, mature-onset diabetes, obesity, colon cancer and probably breast cancer.

4 It makes you feel good by improving your mood and mental health and reducing depression and anxiety.

5 It combats stress and helps you sleep well. But avoid strenuous activity before bed, as it may disrupt sleep. A gentle walk is fine.

6 Exercise improves your posture (so you look slimmer).

7 Combined with healthy eating it gives you more energy and improves your stamina so you can keep going for longer without feeling tired.

8 It helps build denser bones, preventing osteoporosis (which leads to bone fractures and breaks, particularly among women over 50).

9 It improves physical strength and flexibility so you can do everyday tasks, such as carrying and lifting, without getting so tired.

10 It improves the health of people who already suffer from heart disease, high blood pressure, mild depression, raised blood cholesterol or anxiety.

11 Gentle, regular exercise keeps older people mobile and helps them retain their independence. It may also help improve their memory.

12 Exercise also helps your immune system produce more white blood cells to fight infections. But too much exercise reduces them – so don't go mad!

Choose your activities carefully

Be realistic about how much you can achieve. For instance, don't join the Early Risers Swimming Club if you know there's no way you can get to the pool between 6.30 and 7.30 am! Don't book a fitness class if it is going to be a real rush to get to it. In other words, don't set yourself impossible targets – or you will become demotivated.

Try to choose activities that you – and family or friends – will enjoy. Find something you think will be fun or that will make you new friends or develop your interests. Vary your activities so you don't get bored.

Take it one step at a time

Start gently and build up slowly, particularly if you haven't been active for some time. Remember that any activity is better than none. And little changes can make big differences. If 30 minutes, five days a week, is too daunting, try 15 minutes, then two lots of 15 minutes a few times a week, and build up from there. The quick work out option on the *Fighting Fat, Fighting Fit* video will give you around 15 minutes' moderate activity. But stick to the eventual goal of half an hour a day.

Invest in suitable shoes and clothing once you have discovered which activity you prefer and are most likely to stick with. You don't need to go for expensive brands – ask the experts in specialist shops for advice.

It's never too late to start

It's never too late to become more active. Men who take up exercise in their retirement cut their risk of dying from heart disease over the next four years by a third.

However, if you have not exercised before, or you are a man over 40 or a woman over 50 and plan to do strenuous exercise, check first with your GP, and have a proper fitness assessment. You can then have a programme of suitable exercise worked out for you at a local authority class or private club. If you have any health problems (such as high blood pressure, back problems or joint pains) or you are recovering from an operation/illness, it is safest to check with your GP before you start.

★ ★

★ Already going for it

'I feel it is very important to keep fit. I play golf and tennis and swim regularly.'

BBC Radio 2 presenter **ED STEWART** clearly enjoys exercise – and golf, tennis and swimming are a good combination, providing aerobic exercise, stretching muscles and counteracting the effects of stress.

ED STEWART
Height: 1.85 metres (6'1")
Weight: 14 stone *Age:* 50+VAT

★ ★ ★ ★ ★ ★ ★ ★ ★ ★ ★ ★ ★ ★ ★

Facts

How much exercise should different age groups aim for?

Age (men and women)	Target number of 20 minute activity sessions in a four-week period
16–34	12 or more sessions of vigorous activity
35–54	12 or more sessions of activity, mixing moderate and vigorous
55–74	12 or more sessions of moderate activity

Moving on — to more vigorous activity

If you have built up to a level of fitness where you want to go further then it is time to take more vigorous activity. Or, if you already enjoy aerobic exercise and can continue safely, carry on!

The ideal is either five periods of moderate activity a week and/or three periods of vigorous activity. A combination of both types adds variety and interest to your activity regime.

What is vigorous activity?

Vigorous activity is aerobic activity which makes you feel out-of-breath and sweaty. Examples include:

- hill walking at a brisk pace
- squash
- running

- football
- tennis
- aerobics
- cycling

- occupations that involve frequent climbing, lifting or carrying heavy loads
- The *Fighting Fat, Fighting Fit* video includes 20 minutes of vigorous activity

How can you do vigorous exercise safely?

The first step is to work out your theoretical maximum heart rate (MHR) for aerobic exercise. To do this, you have to subtract your age in years from 220. This gives you the maximum heart rate, in beats per minute, for aerobic exercise which increases cardiovascular (heart) fitness.

Now measure your actual heart rate during aerobic exercise by taking your pulse at your neck or wrist. Count the number of beats per minute — or per 15 seconds and multiply by four.

To start with, you should exercise to 50 per cent MHR. Moderate activity is 40–60 per cent, vigorous activity is 60–80 per cent. Or check out the Rate of Perceived Exercise (RPE) chart, another method of measuring the intensity of your activity level, shown in the *Fighting Fat, Fighting Fit* video.

Parents can make families fitter

Getting fit as a family will benefit everyone. Exercise, combined with a balanced diet, will help prevent health problems for the next generation.

At present, by the age of 16, the average child in the UK will have eaten his/her own bodyweight in surplus fat. Coupled with that, children (like most of their parents) are not taking enough exercise. A child with two obese parents has a 70 per cent chance of becoming obese (compared to less than 20 per cent among children of lean parents).

Easy ways to be a more active family

- Twenty years ago, three out of four children walked or cycled to school. Now only around one in five does so. Try to find safe ways for children to walk or cycle more, at least some days each week.
- If this is not possible, try to find ways of replacing that activity. Go for family cycle rides (more children have cycles now, but use them less than previously) or walks. Show your children that being active is an enjoyable part of life.
- Play football/handball/volleyball with your children. Or join them on their roller blades in the park.
- Go for a day's hiking.
- If you have to ferry children to school sport activities, get more involved yourself. Become one of the coaches, run the line, be a referee, train alongside the team to encourage them!
- Make your family holidays more active. Holidays based around activities such as skiing and water sports may seem expensive. But if they are the main holiday of the year they need not be any more expensive than other holidays.
- Take more active holidays in the UK during the summer when the weather should be kinder to outdoor pursuits. Some holidays (such as rambling, guided walking/trekking, working holidays on farms or with organizations such as the National Trust building dry-stone walls or restoring buildings) combine activity with fresh air and friendship. Conservation groups offer accommodation and meals in return for 'work' in a pleasant outdoor environment where new skills can be learned. These are all worth considering.

Polishing off the pounds

Doing housework with attitude can improve your heart-lung fitness. If you know a bit about working out, and you are mindful of your posture, you can make your housework routine into an effective exercise regime. Slow movements down and focus on muscle control to tone muscles:

- Instead of bending to pick things up, or to load and unload the washing machine or dishwasher, use squats to tone bottoms and thighs.
- Work trunk twists and turns into wiping surfaces, and upper arm rotations/flexes into dusting/window cleaning to tone triceps and biceps.
- Lunges and side leg raises while vacuuming tone inner thighs/calves.
- A bit of carpet beating, scrubbing and running up and down stairs to tidy up will all do wonders for weight loss and maintenance.
- Do your abdominal (tummy) exercises as you lie exhausted on the living room floor, waiting for the kettle to boil!

★ ★

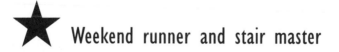 ## Weekend runner and stair master

'I run 2 miles at the weekends. I do it first thing in the morning before I do anything else. I can't bear to exercise later in the day because it's such a drag getting clean again!

'My apartment building has a pool in it so I try to swim about twice a week, if possible. I live in a warehouse which has lots of stairs and that's a great bonus for exercise!'

With regular running, swimming and walking up and down stairs, BBC Radio 2 presenter Sarah does very well for aerobic exercise. She might enjoy doing some muscle-stretching exercise (such as yoga) as well.

SARAH KENNEDY
Height: 1.62 metres (5'4")
Weight: slim Age: 40s

★ ★ ★ ★ ★ ★ ★ ★ ★ ★ ★ ★ ★ ★ ★ ★ ★

★ ★

★ Running round after children does not keep you fit ...

*'It's nonsense that running round after children keeps you fit.
They just stop you sleeping and give you backache, which is not
the same thing!*

*'At university I was a runner and I used to go to the gym
regularly until six years ago when our first child was born. Now
I swim on Sundays but not to keep fit as I have the children
with me. I try to run at weekends and think I should start doing
some exercise properly now.*

*'My wife Linda did yoga during her last pregnancy. I tried some
classes with her and it was great.'*

BBC Radio 2 presenter Richard is quite right about this – it's
one of life's great myths! And it can be hard to fit in exercise
between the demands of work and children. But swimming
and yoga are both good ways to ease back into exercise after a
break, letting you stretch
your muscles gradually
and go at your own pace.

RICHARD ALLINSON
Height: 1.78 metres (5'10")
Weight: 11 stone Age: 40

★ ★ ★ ★ ★ ★ ★ ★ ★ ★ ★ ★ ★ ★ ★

On your bike

Cycling is a good option if you are overweight and are discouraged by
the initial discomfort of jogging or walking (which you can come back
to later). Cycling is not weight-bearing so it is less likely to damage
joints than running. You can start slowly and gradually build up. Just a
20 minute cycle ride a day is a great help towards fitness.

Buy a crash helmet (and a mask in some cities) and cycle to work – it
will save you money and protect the environment. And in large cities
where traffic is heavy it will be much quicker – an 8km (5 mile) journey

can take 35 minutes by bike, 45 by car or train or one hour by bus. For comfort, make sure you choose the right bike for your build and get advice from a specialist retailer, who will also sell secondhand bikes. Get the right clothes, too – not necessarily Lycra shorts! You need clothes to keep out the rain and to cover you so you don't get cold and stiff.

Walking – the best exercise

It may be millions of years since man took his first steps, but walking is still the easiest, most convenient form of exercise. Walking costs nothing, can be done by just about anyone, helps you feel good and relieves tension. It strengthens the heart, muscles and bones, and helps loosen up stiff joints. It improves circulation – and even inspires creative thinking!

★ ★

★ I wish I enjoyed walking more

'I am extremely lazy and only walk when I have to. Sometimes I play tennis or swim in the summer. I wish I did enjoy walking more. It's really only if I am in pleasant surroundings that I attempt a stroll.'

David is typical of the majority of people in the UK. Sadly, playing the odd game of tennis or going for the occasional stroll isn't really enough to benefit your health. The main point is regularity – a daily 20 minute walk to the shops will do you a lot more good than taking strenuous exercise once in a blue moon. You may have to force yourself at first – especially if you lead a busy life like BBC Radio 2 presenter David – but the more you walk, the easier you'll find it, and the more you'll enjoy it ...

DAVID JACOBS
Height: 1.78 metres (5'10")
Weight: 76kg (12 stone) *Age:* 72

★ ★ ★ ★ ★ ★ ★ ★ ★ ★ ★ ★ ★ ★ ★

Getting started with walking

You do not have to do any special stretching, bouncing or other contortions to warm up for walking. Simply walk at a slowish pace for five to eight minutes to increase circulation and breathing. This also warms up the muscles that are going to be worked out and that could be damaged if you started exercising while they are cold.

After five to eight minutes, speed up to a pace you enjoy. Most walkers cruise comfortably at 5.6km (3½ miles) an hour – the speed at which the body was designed to walk. You will even burn off fat if you keep on walking at that speed for 30 minutes every day. However, if you want to train your heart and go in for a little cardiovascular conditioning, you can step up the pace on some days to a brisk walk.

Doing walks at different paces also adds variety and interest, as does varying the route. Try to find a low step or wall 15–20cm (6–8 inches) high and slowly step up and down for 5 minutes, then continue walking. Swing your arms and watch your posture. Focus on using your legs and buttocks as you stride and pull in your tummy and back muscles.

To prevent foot problems, regular walkers should invest in some well-cushioned walking shoes, or make sure that there is at least a thumb's width of space in front of the toes. Dust your feet with powder before walking and moisturize your feet before bed. Wear socks with a high cotton or wool content. If you are doing a day's hiking give your feet a 'breather' during the day by taking off your boots and socks. Change your socks midway for extra comfort.

When not to exercise

Do not exercise vigorously if you are unwell or recovering from a viral illness such as a cold or if you are taking painkillers. Stop straight away if you ever experience pain in the chest, neck or upper left arm, joint pain, dizziness or faintness, severe breathlessness, or exhaustion.

Seven bad reasons for not being active

It's time to let go of all those excuses that have, until now, stopped you benefiting from being active.

1 I don't have time to go to a health club or class Taking enough exercise does not have to take that much time – it can be built into your everyday life. For example, you can walk or cycle instead of using the car, bus or train. You can use the stairs instead of the lift. Even housework can help (see page 91).

2 I'm too tired after work In fact, being more active raises your energy level. But if you do find a particular time of the day more difficult then try to build in your activity session when your energy levels are highest.

3 I hate sport You don't have to do sport to be fit. Walking, cleaning the car or cleaning windows, using the stairs, riding a bike, gardening, dancing are all sport-free exercise zones!

4 I look fat in a leotard/swimsuit You don't have to wear a leotard to go to your local gym. Many gyms set aside specific women-only times and have T-shirt only policies. A T-shirt and leggings or baggy bottoms can look just as good as a leotard and can be equally trendy. However, if you still feel unhappy about visiting a gym, the *Fighting Fat, Fighting Fit* video is an excellent way of getting started and, of course, it has the added advantage that you can do all the exercises in the privacy of your own home. Or go to your local pool on ladies/gents night/afternoon.

5 I can't afford it Walking is great – and it's free.

6 I have back pain Regular exercise will strengthen the muscles that support your back. Seek advice from a physiotherapist or other qualified person on what exercises to do. Swimming and cycling are useful for people with back pain. But if you swim breast-stroke don't keep your head out of the water all the time as this strains the neck.

7 I have arthritis Arthritis can be eased by exercises that keep the muscles and joints working. Low-impact exercise, such as swimming, does not put any stress on the joints. Stretching and strengthening exercises are also good.

If you still think you don't have time for exercise...

Remember, over time, it is your everyday habits that define your fitness, weight and body composition and the way you look and feel. Even if the most you can do is a three-minute walk after every meal it is still worth it, because it amounts to 1.8kg (4lb) less body fat a year. Two flights of stairs a day burns off 225g (8oz) body fat in a year. And so on ... so stay active.

FIGHTING FAT, FIGHTING FIT
SLIMMING
PLAN

If you answered 'Yes' to the question 'Do I need to lose weight?' on page 40, give the *Fighting Fat, Fighting Fit* Slimming Plan a try.

The women's plan is based on 1200 calories a day and the men's is based on 1800 calories per day. Although many slimming diets for women provide 1000 calories a day or less, it is not necessary to eat as little as that to lose weight. In fact, such diets can make fat loss more difficult because they lead to loss of lean (muscle) tissue, which the body burns because it is not receiving enough food for energy.

This is why the *Fighting Fat, Fighting Fit* Slimming Plan is not a crash diet. There is absolutely no point going on a slimming diet that you cannot live with and that doesn't help you change the way you eat – permanently.

The *Fighting Fat, Fighting Fit* Slimming Plan is a gradual weight loss plan because it has been shown that weight lost more slowly is weight less likely to be regained.

In fact, you can even lose weight on the *Fighting Fat, Fighting Fit* Healthy Eating Plan (see page 119) if you need to. But cutting down by about 750 calories per day on normal eating, which is what the *Fighting Fat, Fighting Fit* Slimming Plan does, will make your weight loss slightly quicker.

Although you will be reducing the amount you eat while following the slimming plan, the beauty is that it allows you to eat 'normally'. It will not leave you feeling exhausted or irritable because you will not be hungry and undernourished. And because your body will be receiving the energy it needs, you are far less likely to be tempted to binge on fatty, sugary snacks.

There are none of the nasty side-effects associated with stressful, very low-calorie dieting, and you will not be burning off valuable muscle in order to keep your body ticking over. This is important because you need to have enough energy to continue to be active while you lose weight. Physical activity (see Chapter 4) tones, firms and shapes muscles to bring about the body changes that all slimmers want to see.

How the Slimming Plan works

Both the slimming plan for men and the one for women include three meals a day, plus a variety of snacks.

You can follow the *Fighting Fat, Fighting Fit* Slimming Plan for two weeks, three weeks or four weeks. Although it is not very low in calories, after four weeks it is advisable to increase the amount of food you eat to meet the average daily calorie requirement for men (2550) and women (1940). To do this, you can move on to the *Fighting Fat, Fighting Fit* Healthy Eating Plan (see page 119).

How much weight will you lose?

Assuming your body uses an average 2000 calories a day if you are a woman or 2550 if you are a man, then after a week on the *Fighting Fat, Fighting Fit* Slimming Plan you will have lost more than 5000 calories, the equivalent of more than 0.5kg or nearly 1½lb fat.

Add to that the usual water and glycogen (stored energy) loss that occurs during the first week of slimming and the amount could go up to around 3kg (6½lb) weight loss.

After the first week you can expect to lose a further 0.5kg (1½lb) fat a week – and more if you increase the amount of physical activity you take.

So, in a month you could lose 5–6kg (11–14lb). And because you will be losing the weight at a moderate – but effective – speed, it should stay off permanently, as long as you continue following the *Fighting Fat, Fighting Fit* healthy eating guidelines afterwards. Achieving this weight loss on 1200 or 1800 calories a day is also the least painful way to lose weight.

Should you ever feel the need to return to the *Fighting Fat, Fighting Fit* Slimming Plan, it is safe to do so. But if you just wish to maintain your weight loss you can follow the *Fighting Fat, Fighting Fit* Healthy Eating Plan.

Step up the action

To look and feel even better, you will need to improve your muscle tone and general level of fitness through activity (see Chapter 4). Whatever your age it is never too late to start. But the best way is to be active early in life and to continue regularly through middle age and into old age.

Choose the meals that suit you

There is a free choice from an extensive list of breakfasts, lunches and snacks. And the highlight of the day is a main meal built around one of Ainsley Harriott's fabulous recipes (see page 152). There is no hocus-pocus in this eating programme that forces you to eat particular foods or meals at specific times of the day. With the *Fighting Fat, Fighting Fit* Slimming Plan you can eat your main meal for lunch or for dinner – whichever suits you best.

Although you can choose, within limits, what you want to eat, nutritionally the wisest approach is to eat as wide a variety of foods as possible. This will allow you to enjoy a wide variety of nutrients from different foods. The many different flavours and tastes will also stop you noticing any reduction in the quantity of food.

For example, if your favourite breakfast is Weetabix and your favourite lunch is beef sandwiches, try not to eat them to the exclusion of other foods. Take the opportunity this eating plan offers to be a bit more adventurous. And, most importantly, enjoy your food and the feast of flavours provided by Ainsley's recipes.

General guidelines

The general rules of the slimming plan are:

- No spread on bread or potatoes.
- Eat only one serving of a recipe unless otherwise stated.
- 'Salad' means any combination of the following: green leaves, herbs, tomatoes, cucumber, radish, chicory, peppers, fennel, celery, beetroot, carrot, onion.
- Salads are served without dressing.
- No spread on the bread in sandwiches.
- 'Free choice of vegetables' refers to boiled or steamed green vegetables or carrots or similar (not fried, battered or chips!).
- Milk is skimmed and the quantity used on breakfast cereal is 125ml (4fl oz).
- Fruit juices are unsweetened. The quantity for fruit juice and other drinks in the eating plans and snacks is 125ml (4fl oz).
- Alcoholic drinks are included in the plan. Remember that any additional alcoholic drinks you have will add extra calories to the plan. The quantity of wine is 125ml (4fl oz) per glass.
- The quantity of breakfast cereal is 40g (1½oz).
- Bread (and toast) is from a wholemeal (preferably), medium-sliced large loaf.
- Yoghurts are low-fat and in small tubs – 125g (4½oz).
- Baked potatoes are medium sized – 180g (6½oz).

Drinks

It is recommended that you drink plenty of liquid each day – at least 8 cups or 1.5 litres (2¾ pints), preferably water, or other calorie-free or low-calorie drinks that you enjoy. Limit tea and coffee to 3–4 cups a day and use only a small amount of skimmed milk, or drink them without milk.

The Fighting Fat, Fighting Fit Slimming Plan for Women

1200
CALORIES

Three meals a day are included in this 1200-calorie plan. You can also enjoy a range of snacks. Choose one snack daily from list A (see p. 106) or two from list B (see p. 107).

Breakfast

Choose one of the following breakfasts each day:

- Unsweetened fruit juice
- 2 Weetabix with milk

OR ———

- Cornflakes with milk

OR ———

- Generous 25g (1oz) muesli
- 1 natural or vanilla yoghurt

OR ———

- Porridge – made with 25g (1oz) porridge oats, 200ml (⅓ pint) skimmed milk and 1 teaspoon sugar or syrup

OR ———

- ½ grapefruit with 4 ready-to-eat prunes
- 1 slice toast, 1 teaspoon butter, 1 teaspoon marmalade

OR ———

- Fruit juice
- 2 crispbread, 1 teaspoon butter, 2 teaspoons marmalade or jam

OR ———

- 1 boiled egg
- 1 slice wholemeal toast, 1 teaspoon butter

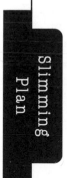
Slimming Plan

continued...

Lunch

Choose one of the following lunches each day:

- Tuna sandwiches – made with 2 slices bread filled with 75g (2¾oz) tuna canned in oil (drained), ¼ green pepper (seeded and chopped), 40g (1½oz) cooked sweetcorn kernels, 40g (1½oz) cooked kidney beans, dash of Tabasco (hot pepper sauce)
- 1 piece of fruit

OR ———————

- ½ carton soup of choice (not vichyssoise or other creamy soup)
- Wholemeal roll, 1 teaspoon butter
- 1 fruit yoghurt

OR ———————

- 2 taco shells filled with unlimited salad, 35g (1¼oz) grated Cheddar-type cheese, 55g (2oz) canned beans

OR ———————

- Ready meal of your choice, of not more than 350 calories, from a range of calorie-counted meals.

OR ———————

- 75g (3oz) reduced-fat hummus, 2 crispbreads or 2 rice cakes
- 1 piece of fruit

OR ———————

- Egg sandwiches – made with 2 slices bread filled with 1 hard-boiled egg mashed with 1 tablespoon low-calorie mayonnaise, seasoning and 25g (1oz) watercress (chopped)
- 1 piece of fruit

OR ———————

continued...

Slimming Plan

- Cheese on toast – made with 2 slices bread, 25g (1oz) thinly pared cheese (a job easily done with a cheese plane), topped with 1 sliced tomato and served with watercress

Dinner

Choose one of the following dinners each day:

- Fuzzyless Jerk Chicken (see p. 153)
- Ainsley's Ultimate Creole Cabbage Salad (see p. 154)
- ½ serving Peppy's Jamaican Rice and Peas (see p. 155)

OR ———

- 2 servings Melintzanosalata with Cherry Tomato Sticks (see p. 156)
- Garlic Pitta Fingers (see p. 157)

OR ———

- 1½ servings Sweet Chilli King Prawns (see p. 158)
- 150g (5½oz) or 4 heaped tablespoons boiled or steamed rice
- 1 mixed salad

OR ———

- 2 servings Cor! Puy Lentil, Red Onion and Sun-dried Tomato Salad (see p. 159)
- Individual or mini pitta bread

OR ———

- Crispy Baton Bacon Potato Cakes (see p. 160)
- 110g (3½oz) broccoli
- 175g (6oz) baked beans
- 1 fruit yoghurt

OR ———

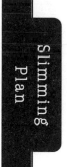

Slimming Plan

continued...

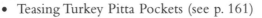

- Teasing Turkey Pitta Pockets (see p. 161)
- Individual meringue nest filled with 90g (3¼oz) fresh fruit compote

  OR ───────

- Fab Haddie and Gooey Egg (see p. 162)
- 110g (3½oz) broccoli
- 175g (6oz) new potatoes, boiled or steamed
- 2 tablespoons peas
- Individual summer fruit pudding

  OR ───────

- Chargrilled Pineapple Chicken Kiss-Kiss (see p. 163)
- Peppy's Jamaican Rice and Peas (see p. 155)
- 110g (3½oz) broccoli or mixed salad

  OR ───────

- Wicked Wine-steamed Mussels (see p. 164)
- 15cm (6 inch) French stick
- Mixed salad

  OR ───────

- Cheesy Cherry Tom Potato Omelette (see p. 165)
- Bread roll
- Orange fruit salad – made with ½ mango, 1 orange, ½ banana

  OR ───────

- Down-in-a-Flash Pumpkin and Potato Soup (see p. 166)
- Bread roll
- Red fruit salad – made with 55g (2oz) each strawberries, raspberries, cherries, 200g (7oz) watermelon

  OR ───────

Slimming Plan

continued...

- Simply Smokin' Paella (see p. 167)
- Ainsley suggests a glass of Rioja – cheers!
- 1 low-fat fruit fool

OR ———

- Plantain, Pumpkin and Chickpea Curry (see p. 168) – although the recipe says 'serves four', in this plan you should eat only one-sixth, not a quarter of the total recipe
- 115g (4 oz) or 3 tablespoons boiled or steamed rice
- Baked peach – made with 1 peach, halved and stoned, and filled with 1 tablespoon low-fat soft white cheese mixed with 1 large ratafia or amaretti biscuit, crushed, and 1 drop almond essence; grill for five minutes

OR ———

- Spicy, Sunny Savoy Cabbage with Bacon and Ginger (see p. 169)
- Baked potato, 2 teaspoons low-fat spread
- 1 piece of fruit

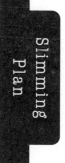

Slimming Plan

continued...

Snack list A

- 1 large banana
- 1 raw lychee
- 1 handful raisins or sultanas – 40g (1½oz)
- 2 reduced-fat fig rolls
- Small chocolate eclair
- Coconut macaroon
- Some leading brands of mini cakes (check labels for calorie content)
- Lower-calorie cereal/fruit bars
- Low-fat fruit fools and mousses
- 2 cheese spread triangles
- 25g (1oz) chocolate raisins
- Small teacake
- Small shop-bought pancakes
- 1 slice malt loaf, unspread
- 1 slice wholemeal toast with 1 teaspoon low-fat spread
- Diet cake bar
- 25g (1oz) Twiglets
- 25g (1oz) plain or caramel/sugar-coated popcorn
- Mini cheeses (check label for calorie content)

There are other low-calorie family-size cakes available in supermarkets and grocers including: 95–96 per cent fat-free Danish pastries, brownies, muffins, chocolate cake, fruit cake, orange cake, Madeira cake. Check the nutrition label on the packet for 100 calorie portion size.

continued...

Snack list B

- 1 large glass semi-skimmed milk – 200ml (7fl oz)
- 1 large glass unsweetened orange juice – 250ml (9fl oz)
- Apple
- 4–5 apricots
- 20 cherries
- 2 medium clementines (or other easy peelers, e.g. mandarins, satsumas)
- 3 fresh dates
- 1 dried date
- 2 fresh figs
- 1 dried fig
- 1 small bunch seedless grapes (about 20 grapes) – 100g (3½oz)
- 2 small kiwi fruit
- 1 peach or nectarine
- 1 pear
- 2½ plums
- Rice cake
- Fig roll
- Jaffa cake
- 2 breadsticks (grissini)
- 3 matzos
- Poppadom
- Mini *pain au raisin*
- Mini ring doughnut

The Fighting Fat, Fighting Fit Slimming Plan for Men

1800 CALORIES

Three meals a day are included in this 1800-calorie plan, plus snacks – one from list C (see p. 113), or two from list A (see p. 106), or four from list B (see p. 107).

Breakfast

Choose a double portion of any of the women's 1200-calorie breakfasts (see p. 101) or choose one of the following each day:

- 1 grilled sausage
- 1 egg fried in non-stick pan without added fat, or poached or boiled
- 1 grilled tomato
- 55g (2oz) poached mushrooms
- 2 slices toast, 2 teaspoons low-fat spread

OR ———

- 2 Shredded Wheat with milk and 1 sliced medium banana
- 1 slice toast, 1 teaspoon low-fat spread, 2 teaspoons jam

OR ———

- 80g (3oz) large portion of Alpen (the version with no added sugar) with 200ml (⅓ pint) skimmed milk
- Fruit juice

OR ———

- BLT – made with 2 slices bread, 2 grilled lean rashers of back bacon, 1 tomato, a few lettuce leaves

OR ———

- Porridge (see p. 101)
- 1 × 175g (6oz) medium kipper
- Orange juice

continued...

OR ———————

- 175g (6oz) poached smoked haddock
- 1 poached egg
- 2 slices toast, 2 teaspoons low-fat spread

Lunch

Choose one of the following lunches each day:

- Baked potato
- 150g (5½oz) chilli con carne
- Salad
- 1 piece of fruit

  OR ———————

- 150g (5½oz) grilled lean pork loin chop
- 125g (4½oz) each of carrots and cabbage
- 2 tablespoons peas

  OR ———————

- 225g (8oz) cauliflower cheese (individual 300 calorie ready-meal size)
- 4 tablespoons peas
- 1 beefsteak tomato, grilled
- 1 banana

  OR ———————

- 3 fish fingers, grilled
- 175g (6oz) oven chips (medium portion)
- 2 tablespoons peas

  OR ———————

- Roast beef salad sandwich
- 1 packet crisps
- 1 piece of fruit

  OR ———————

continued...

Slimming
Plan

- Baked potato
- Mixed salad
- ½ avocado filled with 115g (4oz) shelled cooked prawns mixed with 1 tablespoon reduced-calorie mayonnaise and 1 teaspoon tomato ketchup

OR ————

- Individual 12.5–17.5cm (5–7 inch) ham and mushroom pizza or ½ large frozen/takeaway pizza
- Mixed salad
- Orange juice

OR ————

- 300g (10½oz) pasta and vegetable salad (approximately 300 calories)

OR ————

- Ham salad – made with 2 slices lean roast ham, 115g (4oz) low-calorie coleslaw, mixed salad, 115g (4oz) potato salad
- Orange juice

Dinner

Choose one of the following dinners each day:

- Fuzzyless Jerk Chicken (see p. 153)
- Ainsley's Ultimate Creole Cabbage Salad (see p. 154)
- Peppy's Jamaican Rice and Peas (see p. 155)

OR ————

- 2 servings Melintzanosalata with Cherry Tomato Sticks (see p. 156)
- Garlic Pitta Fingers (see p. 157)
- 150g (5½oz) pot or can low-fat rice pudding, with 60g (2¼oz) raspberries stirred in

OR ————

continued...

1800 CALORIES

- 2 servings Sweet Chilli King Prawns (see p. 158)
- Peppy's Jamaican Rice and Peas (see p. 155)

  OR ———

- 2 servings Cor! Puy Lentil, Onion and Sun-dried Tomato Salad (see p. 159)
- 1 large pitta bread

  OR ———

- Crispy Baton Bacon Potato Cakes (see p. 160)
- 115g (4oz) broccoli
- 1 poached egg
- 200g (7oz) baked beans (half a large can)
- 2 slices bread

  OR ———

- 1½ servings Teasing Turkey Pitta Pockets (see p. 161)
- 1 fruit yoghurt

  OR ———

- Fab Haddie and Gooey Egg (see p. 162)
- 115g (4oz) broccoli
- 175g (6oz) new potatoes, boiled or steamed
- 2 tablespoons peas
- 115g (4oz) apple strudel

  OR ———

- Chargrilled Pineapple Chicken Kiss-Kiss (see p. 163)
- 1½ servings Peppy's Jamaican Rice and Peas (see p. 155)
- 115g (4oz) broccoli
- 80g (3oz) sweetcorn

  OR ———

Slimming Plan

continued...

1800 CALORIES

- Salade Niçoise – made with lettuce, tomato, 55g (2oz) cold, cooked French beans, 1 hard-boiled egg, 4 anchovy fillets, 4 black olives
- Wicked Wine-steamed Mussels (see p. 164)
- 15cm (6 inch) French stick

OR ————

- Avocado Salad – made with lettuce, celery, ½ avocado, 25g (1oz) walnuts, ½ apple
- Cheesy Cherry Tom Potato Omelette (see p. 165)
- Bread roll

OR ————

- Down-in-a-Flash Pumpkin and Potato Soup (see p. 166)
- Toasted sandwich – made with 2 slices bread, 1 slice ham, 25g (1oz) Cheddar
- Mixed salad

OR ————

- 1½ servings Simply Smokin Paella (see p. 167)
- Ainsley suggests a glass of Rioja – cheers!
- 1 piece of fruit

OR ————

- Plantain, Pumpkin and Chickpea Curry (see p. 168)
- Peppy's Jamaican Rice and Peas (see p. 155)
- Crème caramel (chilled dessert)

OR ————

- Spicy, Sunny Savoy Cabbage with Bacon and Ginger (see p. 169)
- 1 medium baked potato

continued...

Slimming Plan

Snack list C

- Wholemeal hot cross bun, spiced fruited bun or currant bun
- Wholemeal fruit scone and either 2 teaspoons low-fat spread or 2 teaspoons preserve
- 200ml (½ pint) chocolate milk or hot chocolate
- Bath bun
- 1 packet crisps and an apple
- Granary roll spread thinly with black olive pâté or tapenade
- 1 small bag roasted, salted nuts – 25g (1oz)
- 1 bagel
- ½ bagel spread with 2 tablespoons low-fat soft white cheese and 25g (1oz) smoked salmon
- 3–4 dried dates
- 1 samosa
- 75g (3oz) dried ready-to-eat pears, apricots or peaches
- Cup of soup and bread roll
- 3–4 grilled fish fingers
- Small jacket potato with 25g (1oz) cottage cheese
- 2 slices wholemeal toast with 2 teaspoons low-fat spread
- Scrambled egg on 1 slice toast

Snack list C

Slim-line eating out

Many people who are slimming think that if they take a day off from their eating plan, or go out for a meal, they have 'blown it'. This is particularly common on very low-calorie diets that leave slimmers undernourished and ravenous. Such diets put slimmers under the kind of pressure that can lead to binges.

However, with *Fighting Fat, Fighting Fit,* there is no harm at all in departing from the calorie-counted plan. Simply pick up where you left off the next day. Of course your weight loss will be a little slower but, as we keep saying, weight lost more gradually is weight that is far less likely to be regained.

Feeling secure enough about your eating habits to let go of your slimming plan for a day is also important because this is the basis of normal healthy eating for the future. Once you have reached a healthy weight, you will want to eat in the same way as people who are not slimming. And that means enjoying a natural balance between 'normal' healthy eating most of the time and being able to fully enjoy the feasting associated with special occasions. If you need to you can always eat a little less for a couple of days before or after a special (eating) occasion.

Desk snacks

If you are prone to 'snack attacks' it is worth keeping some nibbles in your desk drawer – that way you won't have to go and buy something in the canteen at work or at the local corner shop. The exercise may do you good but you will inevitably be faced with a wide range of sugary confectionery and fatty savoury snacks. Better to go shopping when you are not ravenous ... so snack first.

Snack suggestions can be taken from the previous lists, which include fresh fruit. In addition, some more snack ideas include snack-size packs of prunes or other dried fruit mixtures, crunchy breakfast cereal, pots of cereal with milk and a spoon included in the lid, lower-fat pretzels or lower-fat, unsalted crisps, crispbread, breadsticks and small quantities of nuts.

Some sample menus

Here are some sample daily menus showing how you can adapt the slimming plan to your own lifestyle.

Vegetarian mother at home

Breakfast

- ½ grapefruit with 4 ready-to-eat prunes
- 1 slice toast, 1 teaspoon butter, 1 teaspoon marmalade

Lunch

- ½ carton soup of choice (not vichyssoise or other creamy soup)
- Wholemeal roll, 1 teaspoon butter
- 1 fruit yoghurt

Dinner

- Plantain, Pumpkin and Chickpea Curry (see p. 168) – although the recipe says 'serves four', in this plan you should eat only one-sixth, not a quarter of the total recipe
- 115g (4oz) or 3 tablespoons boiled or steamed rice

- Baked peach – made with 1 peach, halved and stoned, and filled with 1 tablespoon low-fat soft white cheese mixed with 1 large ratafia, crushed, and 1 drop almond essence; grill for five minutes

Snacks

- Mini *pain au raisin*
- 1 small bunch seedless grapes (about 20 grapes) – 100g (3½oz)

Busy working woman aged up to 50

Breakfast

- Cornflakes with milk

Lunch

- Egg sandwich – made with 2 slices bread filled with 1 hard-boiled egg mashed with 1 tablespoon low-calorie mayonnaise, seasoning and 25g (1oz) chopped watercress
- 1 piece of fruit

Dinner

- Chargrilled Pineapple Chicken Kiss-Kiss (see p. 163)
- Peppy's Jamaican Rice and Peas (see p. 155)
- 110g (3½oz) broccoli or mixed salad

Snacks

- Jaffa cake
- 1 pear

Retired woman at home

Breakfast

- Porridge (see p. 101)

Lunchtime main meal

- Fab Haddie and Gooey Egg (see p. 162)
- 110g (3½oz) broccoli
- 175g (6oz) new potatoes, boiled or steamed
- 2 tablespoons peas
- Individual summer fruit pudding

Supper

- Cheese on toast – made with 2 slices bread, 25g (1oz) thinly pared cheese (a job easily done with a cheese plane), topped with 1 sliced tomato and served with watercress

Snacks

- 1 glass semi-skimmed milk – 200ml (7fl oz)
- 1 apple

Busy working man

Breakfast

- 80g (3oz) large portion of Alpen (the version with no added sugar) with 200ml (⅓ pint) skimmed milk
- Fruit juice

Lunch

- Baked potato, filled with 150g (5½oz) chilli con carne
- Salad
- 1 piece of fruit

Dinner

- 1½ servings Simply Smokin Paella (see p. 167)
- Ainsley suggests a glass of Rioja – cheers!
- 1 piece of fruit

Snacks

- 2 poppadoms
- 95 per cent fat-free Danish pastry

Man at home

Breakfast

- BLT – made with 2 slices bread, 2 grilled lean rashers of back bacon, 1 tomato, a few lettuce leaves

Lunch

- 3 fish fingers, grilled
- 175g (6oz) oven chips (medium portion)
- 2 tablespoons peas

Dinner

- 2 servings Sweet Chilli King Prawns (see p. 158)
- Peppy's Jamaican Rice and Peas (see p. 155)

Snack

- Wholemeal fruit scone and either 2 teaspoons low-fat spread or 2 teaspoons preserve

Retired man at home

Breakfast

- Porridge (see p. 101)
- 1 × 175g (6oz) medium kipper
- Orange juice

Lunchtime main meal

- Crispy Baton Bacon Potato Cakes (see p. 160)
- 115g (4oz) broccoli
- 1 poached egg
- 200g (7oz) baked beans (half a large can)
- 2 slices bread

Supper

- Roast beef salad sandwich
- 1 packet crisps
- 1 piece of fruit

Snack

- 200ml (7fl oz) chocolate milk or hot chocolate, or a Bath bun

HEALTHY EATING PLAN

If you answered 'Yes' to the question 'Do I need to change my eating habits?' on page 40 then the *Fighting Fat, Fighting Fit* Healthy Eating Plan will help you choose foods in the best proportions for healthy eating.

There is one eating plan for women, based on 1940 calories a day, and one for men, based on 2550 calories per day. These amounts will not provide enough energy for people who are very active, but the vast majority of us are relatively sedentary.

The *Fighting Fat, Fighting Fit* Healthy Eating Plan is not a weight loss plan. However, if you habitually ate more calories than you burnt off, or more than the above amounts, then you will lose weight.

You may also find that the foods included in the plan are more nutritious than the foods you normally eat. If this is the case you will benefit from a greater intake of vitamins and minerals which will boost your general health and should, within a couple of months, make you feel less tired and more energetic.

Because the plan is not a slimming diet you can follow it for as long as you like in complete safety. However, we hope you will get a taste for what constitutes well-balanced eating and a feel for the quantity of food that does not lead to weight gain. You can then shop, cook and eat out in your own way without having to follow a plan. The *Fighting Fat, Fighting Fit* Maintenance Plan (see page 136) will help you to do this.

The attraction of this healthy eating plan is that it gives you freedom of choice. You don't have to eat a set meal on a set day of the week – you can build your own meal patterns to suit your lifestyle.

How the Healthy Eating Plan works

Both the healthy eating plan for men and the one for women include three meals a day, plus a variety of snacks.

You can follow the plan for two weeks, three weeks, four weeks or as long as you like. We would recommend a maximum of four weeks, after which you can go off on your own voyage of discovery – perhaps still using some of your favourite recipes and dishes from the eating plan.

Shape the Healthy Eating Plan to suit your lifestyle

There is a free choice on the *Fighting Fat, Fighting Fit* Healthy Eating Plan from an extensive list of breakfasts, lunches and snacks. Highlight of the day is a stunning main meal built around one of Ainsley Harriott's fabulous recipes. Don't worry – you don't have to be a chef to tackle the recipes. Many of the ingredients are familiar but they are all extremely tasty. You can eat your main meal at any time of day – lunchtime or evening, whenever suits you and your family.

Although we all have our personal food likes and dislikes, variety is the key to healthy eating. So try to choose as widely as you can from the foods and meals available on the lists below.

Doing so will ensure that you enjoy a wide variety of nutrients available from different foods because no food contains all the vitamins and minerals we need for health.

Use this healthy eating plan as an opportunity to try new foods and new flavours – and have fun.

General guidelines

Because this is a calorie-counted plan there are a few rules:

- No spread on bread or potatoes.
- Eat only one serving of a recipe unless otherwise stated.
- Salad means any combination of the following: green leaves, herbs, tomatoes, cucumber, radish, chicory, peppers, fennel, celery, beetroot, carrot, onion.
- Salads are served without dressing.

Facts

Physical activity

As you are now feeling inspired to change the way you eat, you might also like to improve your level of fitness. This might mean starting from scratch or building on the activities you already do. However, if you feel you would like to concentrate on one thing at a time, then take it at your own pace, stepping up the action once you are comfortable with your new eating habits. After all, changing eating habits is a major achievement in itself. So, do not worry, it is never too late to start taking, or increasing, physical activity (See chapter 4).

- No spread on the bread in sandwiches.
- 'Free choice of vegetables' refers to boiled or steamed green vegetables or carrots or similar (not fried, battered or chips!).
- Milk is skimmed and the quantity used on breakfast cereal is 125ml (4fl oz).
- Fruit juices are unsweetened. The quantity for fruit juice and other drinks in the plans and snacks is 125ml (4fl oz).
- Alcoholic drinks are included in the plan. Remember that any additional alcoholic drinks you have will add extra calories to the plan. The quantity of wine is 125ml (4fl oz) per glass.
- The quantity of breakfast cereal is 40g (1½oz)
- Bread (and toast) is from a medium-sliced large loaf.
- Yoghurts are low-fat and in small tubs – 125g (4½oz).
- Baked potatoes are medium sized – 180g (6½oz).

Drinks

Drink at least 8 cups or 1.5 litres (2¾ pints) a day. Limit tea and coffee to 3–4 cups.

The Fighting Fat, Fighting Fit Healthy Eating Plan for Women

Three meals a day are included in the 1940-calorie plan, plus snacks. Choose one snack from list C (see p. 113), or two snacks from list A (see p. 106), or four from snack list B (see p. 107).

Breakfast

As for the 1800-calorie slimming plan for men (see p. 108)

Lunch

Choose one of the following lunches each day:

- Sandwich – made with 115g (4oz) ciabatta, filled with 125g (4½oz) reduced-fat mozzarella, 1 sliced tomato, and shredded basil leaves
- Papaya, seeded and filled with 8 sliced strawberries, with lime juice squeezed over to taste

OR ———

- Ainsley's Baked Potato, Pepper and Onion Frittata (see p. 170)
- Fruit salad – made with ½ mango, 1 orange, ½ banana

OR ———

- Ainsley's Chicken Show-Stopper Stir-fry (see p. 171)
- 75g (2¾oz) boiled or steamed noodles
- Orange juice

continued...

Healthy
Eating Plan

OR ————

- Tuna sandwich – made with 2 slices bread, 45g (1¾oz) tuna in oil, drained, 1 tablespoon soft white low-fat cheese, and ¼ green pepper, diced
- 55g (2oz) Twiglets
- 1 piece of fruit

OR ————

- Sardines on toast – made with 1 can sardines in tomato sauce on 2 slices toast
- Watercress and orange salad
- 1 low-fat chocolate mousse

OR ————

- Alternatively, choose any of the lunches from the 1800-calorie slimming plan for men (see p.109) with an additional large piece of fruit or an additional 125ml (4fl oz) unsweetened fruit juice.

Dinner

Choose one of the following dinners each day:

- Munchie Mustard Chicken Escalopes (see p. 172)
- Baked potato
- 1 piece of fruit

OR ————

- Moroccan Spiced Lamb Kebabs (see p. 173)
- Spicy Casablanca Couscous (see p. 174)

OR ————

- Sally's Salmon Steaks with Fresh Basil Sauce (see p. 175)
- 175g (6oz) new potatoes, boiled or steamed

continued...

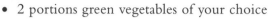

1940
CALORIES

- 2 portions green vegetables of your choice
- 1 fruit yoghurt

  OR ———
- Speckled-eye Squash Stew (see p. 176)
- Individual or mini naan bread
- Blackcurrant brulée – made with 115g (4oz) stewed blackcurrants and 1 teaspoon sugar in a ramekin; top with 3 tablespoons Greek-style natural yoghurt and sprinkle with 2 teaspoons demerara sugar; then put under a preheated hot grill until the sugar melts and bubbles

  OR ———
- Tossed Beansprout Prawn Noodles (see p. 177)
- 55g (2oz) prawn crackers
- Oriental fruit salad – made with 6 lychees, seeded and chopped, with 1 mandarin, segmented

  OR ———
- Cod Kebabs with Aztec Salsa (see p. 178)
- Mixed salad
- Iced Fresh Fruit Platter with Passionfruit Cream (see p. 179)

  OR ———
- Char Sui Lettuce Rolls (see p. 180)
- 200g (7oz) egg-fried rice or 250g (9oz) vegetable chow mein (approximately 300 calories)

  OR ———
- Sinhalese Pasta (see p. 181)

  OR ———
- Cor!! Coriander Lemon Chicken (see p. 182)
- Cool Carrot, Cumin and Lemon Salad (see p. 183)

continued...

Healthy
Eating Plan

OR ———

- Grilled Tuna with Green Lentil Salad (see p. 184)
- 175g (6oz) ratatouille (approximately 100 calories)
- Individual summer fruit pudding

  OR ———

- Red Stripe Linguine with Chestnut Mushrooms and Basil (see p. 185)

  OR ———

- Crunchy Cod and Mash (see p. 187)
- 140g (5oz) apple crumble (approximately 100 calories)
- 125ml (4fl oz) low-fat custard

  OR ———

- Smoked Bacon, Creamy Tomatoes, Peas and Penne Pasta (see p. 188)

  OR ———

- Superb Mackerel with Chilli and Herbs (see p. 189)
- Peppy's Jamaican Rice and Peas (see p. 155)

Healthy
Eating Plan

The Fighting Fat, Fighting Fit Healthy Eating Plan for Men

2550 CALORIES

Three meals a day are included in the 2550-calorie plan. Choose a mid-morning/afternoon snack from list A (see p. 106) or two from list B (see p. 107) or two from the list on page 131. In addition, you can have either one snack from list C (see p. 113) or two snacks from list A, or four snacks from list B.

Breakfast

Double portions from the 1800-calorie slimming plan for men (see p. 108), or choose one of the following breakfasts each day:

- 2 waffles
- 140g (5oz) fresh fruit salad
- Small pot low-fat vanilla yoghurt

  OR ———

- Fruit juice
- 2 pancakes with 2 tablespoons maple syrup and 175g (6oz) blueberries

  OR ———

- 125g (4½oz) low-fat natural yoghurt with 1 teaspoon honey and 4 ready-to-eat prunes
- Blueberry muffin

  OR ———

- Croissant with 4 teaspoons reduced-sugar jam
- Orange juice
- 2 fresh figs
- Cappuccino

  OR ———

continued...

- Orange juice
- *Pain au chocolat*
- 140g (5oz) fresh fruit salad

  OR ─────
- 140g (5oz) kipper
- 1 slice bread
- Orange juice

  OR ─────
- Orange juice
- 40g (1½oz) cornflakes with milk
- Grilled fishcake (approximately 150 calories)

Lunch

Choose one of the following lunches each day:

- Hummus and carrot sandwiches – made with 2 slices wholemeal bread, 55g (2oz) reduced-fat hummus and 1 medium carrot, grated
- 1 packet crisps
- Cereal bar
- 200ml (7fl oz) carton unsweetened fruit juice

  OR ─────
- Ploughman's lunch – made with 150g (5½oz) Granary bread, 50g (1¾oz) Cheddar-type cheese, 1 tablespoon pickle, lettuce, tomato and onion
- 300ml (½ pint) bitter/beer

  OR ─────
- French ploughman's – made with 15cm (6 inch) French stick and 75g (3oz) Camembert
- 175g (6oz) ratatouille (approximately 100 calories)
- 1 glass red wine

Healthy Eating Plan

continued...

2550
CALORIES

Healthy
Eating Plan

OR ———————

- Burger and fries – typical high-street chain quarter-pounder, small fries
- Large orange juice – 250ml (9fl oz)

OR ———————

- Tortillas – made with 2 wheat tortillas, filled with refried beans, and topped with 40g (1½oz) grated cheese
- 50g (1¾oz) guacamole and 50g (1¾oz) salsa, plus chopped onion and tomato
- 330ml (11fl oz) bottle Sol beer

OR ———————

- Beef enchilada (approximately 700 calories)
- 1 piece of fruit

OR ———————

- Triple sandwich pack – typical high street or supermarket pack (approximately 600 calories)
- 200ml (7fl oz) carton fresh pressed apple juice
- Large banana

OR ———————

- Swedish salad – made with 55g (2oz) gravadlax, 85g (3oz) potato salad and mixed green salad
- 1 glass white wine
- 125g (4½oz) cheesecake (approximately 350 calories)

Dinner

Choose one of the following dinners each day:

- Munchie Mustard Chicken Escalopes (see p. 172)
- Large baked potato – 225g (8oz)
- Individual sponge pudding (approximately 350 calories)

continued...

OR ————

- Moroccan Spiced Lamb Kebabs (see p. 173)
- Spicy Casablanca Couscous (see p. 174)
- 2 portions vegetables of your choice
- Individual fruit trifle

OR ————

- Sally's Salmon Steaks with Fresh Basil Sauce (see p. 175)
- 2 portions vegetables of your choice
- 225g (8oz) new potatoes, boiled or steamed
- 140g (5oz) fresh fruit salad
- 2 scoops vanilla ice-cream – 100g (3½oz)
- 1 glass white wine

OR ————

- Speckled-eye Squash Stew (see p. 176)
- Large naan bread
- 95g (3¼oz) pear tart or other fruit tart (approximately 200 calories)

OR ————

- Tossed Beansprout Prawn Noodles (see p. 177)
- 330ml (11fl oz) bottle beer
- Pecan Danish pastry (approximately 400 calories)

OR ————

- gazpacho (approximately 80 calories) with 2 crispbread or crisp rolls
- Cod Kebabs with Aztec Salsa (see p. 178)
- Mixed salad with 2 tablespoons vinaigrette
- Crème caramel with 60g (2¼oz) raspberries
- 1 glass white wine

OR ————

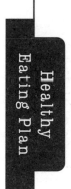

continued...

- 3 prawn toasts
- Char Sui Lettuce Rolls (see p. 180)
- Black cherry gateau (approximately 350 calories)

  OR ————

- Sinhalese Pasta (see p. 181)

  OR ————

- Cor!! Coriander Lemon Chicken (see p. 182)
- Cool Carrot, Cumin and Lemon Salad (see p. 183)
- 200g (7oz) or 5 tablespoons boiled or steamed rice

  OR ————

- Grilled Tuna with Green Lentil Salad (see p. 184)
- 175g (6oz) ratatouille (approximately 100 calories)
- Strawberry gateau (approximately 300 calories)
- Orange juice

  OR ————

- Red Stripe Linguine with Chestnut Mushrooms and Basil (see p. 185)
- Salad with 2 tablespoons vinaigrette

  OR ————

- Pinky Grapefruit, Prawn and Avocado Salad (see p. 186)
- Crunchy Cod and Mash (see p. 187)
- 2 portions vegetables of your choice
- 90g (3¼oz) lemon cheesecake (approximately 300 calories)

  OR ————

- Smoked Bacon, Creamy Tomatoes, Peas and Penne Pasta (see p. 188)

  OR ————

continued...

Healthy
Eating Plan

2550
CALORIES

- Superb Mackerel with Chilli and Herbs (see p. 189)
- Peppy's Jamaican Rice and Peas (see p. 155)
- 115g (4oz) bread and butter pudding (approximately 250 calories)

Snacks

See page 126 for the number of snacks you can have on the 2550-calorie plan.

- Low-fat fruit fool
- Diet chocolate mousse
- Prosciutto (Parma ham) open sandwich – made with 2 slices dark rye crispbread, topped with salad leaves and 2 wafer-thin slices prosciutto with fat cut off
- 2 small scoops frozen yoghurt
- Large oatcake

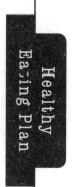

Healthy
Eating Plan

Some sample menus

Here are some sample daily menus showing how you can adapt the healthy eating plan to suit your own lifestyle.

Woman at home

Breakfast

- Orange juice
- 80g (3oz) large portion Alpen (the version with no added sugar) with 200ml (⅓ pint) milk

Lunch

- Chicken Show-Stopper Stir-Fry (see p. 171)
- 75g (2¾oz) boiled or steamed noodles
- Orange juice

Dinner

- Red Stripe Linguine with Chestnut Mushrooms and Basil (see p. 185)

Snacks

- Apple
- 4–5 apricots
- Low-calorie chocolate cake bar

Busy working woman aged up to 50

Breakfast

- 2 Shredded Wheat with milk
- Medium banana
- 1 slice toast, 1 teaspoon low-fat spread, 2 teaspoons jam

Lunch

- Tuna sandwich – made with 2 slices bread, 45g (1¾oz) tuna in oil, drained, 1 tablespoon soft white low-fat cheese, and ¼ green pepper, diced
- 55g (2oz) Twiglets
- 1 piece of fruit

Dinner
- Moroccan Spiced Lamb Kebabs (see p. 173)
- Spicy Casablanca Couscous (see p. 174)

Snacks
- 1 large banana
- 25g (1oz) chocolate raisins

Retired woman at home

Breakfast
Have a double portion of any of the women's 1200-calorie breakfasts (see p. 101), or choose a combination of any two, e.g.:
- 40g (1½oz) cornflakes with 125ml (4fl oz) skimmed milk, 1 boiled egg, 1 slice wholemeal toast, 1 teaspoon butter

Lunch
- Sardines on toast – made with 1 can sardines in tomato sauce and 2 slices toast
- Watercress and orange salad
- 1 low-fat chocolate mousse

Dinner
- Munchie Mustard Chicken Escalopes (see p. 172)
- Baked potato
- 1 piece of fruit

Snacks
- Coconut macaroon
- 3 fresh dates
- 1 glass semi-skimmed milk

Busy working man

Breakfast
- Croissant with 4 teaspoons reduced-sugar jam
- Orange juice

- 2 fresh figs
- Cappuccino

Lunch

- French ploughman's – made with 15cm (6 inch) French stick and 80g (3oz) Camembert
- 175g (6oz) ratatouille (approximately 100 calories)
- 1 glass red wine

Dinner

- Superb Mackerel with Chilli and Herbs (see p. 189)
- Peppy's Jamaican Rice and Peas (see p. 155)
- 115g (4oz) bread and butter pudding (approximately 250 calories)

Snacks

- 1 packet crisps
- Apple

Man at home

Breakfast

- Orange juice
- 40g (1½oz) cornflakes with milk
- Grilled fishcake (approximately 150 calories)

Lunch

- Burger and fries – typical high-street chain quarter-pounder, small fries
- Large orange juice

Dinner

- Tossed Beansprout Prawn Noodles (see p. 177)
- 330ml (11fl oz) bottle beer
- Pecan Danish pastry (approximately 400 calories)

Snacks

- Apple
- 25g (1oz) Twiglets

Retired man at home

Breakfast

- Orange juice
- 1 × 140g (5oz) kipper
- 1 slice bread

Lunch

- Pinky Grapefruit, Prawn and Green Avocado Salad (see p. 186)
- Crunchy Cod and Mash (see p. 187)
- 2 portions vegetables of your choice
- 90g (3¼oz) lemon cheesecake (approximately 300 calories)

Supper

- Swedish salad – made with 55g (2oz) gravadlax, 80g (3oz) potato salad and mixed green salad
- 1 glass white wine,
- 125g (4½oz) cheesecake (approximately 350 calories)

Snacks

- Small teacake
- Medium clementine (or other easy peeler, e.g. mandarin, satsuma)

FIGHTING FAT, FIGHTING FIT
MAINTENANCE PLAN

Whether you have followed the *Fighting Fat, Fighting Fit* Slimming Plan or the Healthy Eating Plan – or both! – we hope that they have helped change the way you eat and that you have enjoyed the experience.

Having reached your desired weight, you can continue to eat the foods you like, in the right proportions, and say goodbye to the vicious circle of crash-dieting followed by binge-eating.

If you have started to become more physically active, as well as changing your eating habits, it will be even easier to maintain your weight loss. Studies have shown that physically active people are more likely to sustain a higher percentage of weight lost through dieting. The good news is that, no matter how unenthusiastic you are about starting to take more exercise, physical activity will automatically improve your mood and make you feel happier about your shape and appearance.

We hope that through following the *Fighting Fat, Fighting Fit* eating plans you have come some way to overcoming your guilt feelings about sugary foods and realizing that unrealistic slimming goals only lead to unhappiness, anxiety and tiredness.

This chapter gives practical advice on maintaining your weight, from changing the foods on your shopping list to changing the way you prepare, cook and serve them. Even if you don't often cook for yourself, but eat out a lot or stay in hotels, there are many ways to gain more control of your food choices.

Eating out

For some people, eating out is the rule rather than the exception. If you frequently eat in canteens, cafés, restaurants or hotels, here are some tips on how to make the best choices from the food available.

Remember, these guidelines are for people who eat out on a *very regular basis*. They are not 'killjoy' rules for birthdays or other celebrations. The whole point of celebratory meals is to enjoy different foods, many of which may be richer than usual. Such occasional feasting is all part of the enjoyment of food and will not ruin or undermine general healthy eating habits.

Aperitifs

Avoid additional alcohol and you will avoid taking in a substantial number of 'empty' non-nutritional calories.

- If you are going to have wine with your meal, you could order the wine to be opened and enjoy a glass ahead of the meal.
- If you are a resident at a hotel you do not need to drink the whole bottle (six glasses) at one meal. Do as they do on the Continent – ask for the wine to be stoppered and held for the next meal.
- And don't overlook half-bottles.
- Or, instead of alcohol, have fruit juices or mineral water for an aperitif - these days they are quite 'socially acceptable' options!
- Avoid crisps, nuts and other salty or fatty savoury snacks before a meal. If you cannot resist snacks, grissini (breadsticks), pretzels and crudités (raw vegetables) are better options.

Starters

- Bread is often offered before a meal – this is a good way to increase your starchy complex carbohydrate intake, especially with speciality breads which are so tasty that they can be enjoyed without added butter.
- Avoid pâtés, meat or fish mousses, fried foods (such as goujons of fish or whitebait) and their high-fat accompaniments such as tartare or other creamy or mayonnaise-based sauces. Avoid 'cream of', or 'creamed soups'.

- Instead, choose smoked salmon or gravadlax which are lower in fat. Or choose clear vegetable soups, consommés, salads or melon.

Main course

- Avoid fried foods, fish or meat in batter, and anything served with creamy or buttery sauces. Avoid fatty meats such as duck.
- Choose lean meat, game, poultry or fish. Opt for grilled (except for fish meunière which is grilled in oodles of butter), or char-grilled dishes.
- Remove any visible fat.

Cheese course

- In general, avoid the cheese course (unless you have not had a starter and you are not having a pudding).
- If you cannot resist cheese, don't accompany it with bread or biscuits.
- And if you do, eat them unbuttered.
- Instead of bread or biscuits, have fruit (pears/grapes) or celery.
- Try lower-fat fresh cheeses (see page 149) with fresh fruits.

Puddings

- Avoid them almost entirely. Starters and main courses are often better value nutritionally than puddings – except for fresh fruit, real fruit sorbet or fruit salad (without the cream).
- Avoid, in particular, pastries, pies, cheesecakes, soufflés, mousses, gateaux, crème brûlée and crème caramel.

Coffee

- Choose black coffee or herb or fruit teas, which are much lower in calories and fat than *caffe latte*, cappuccino, Irish coffee and other coffees flavoured with liqueurs.

Petits fours

- In some restaurants these are so wonderful that they are a 'pudding' in themselves. As a regular diner, you will know in which restaurants to skip pudding and cheese and have coffee and petits fours instead!

- After-dinner mints, truffles, chocolates and liqueurs are one of those extras that regular diners are much better doing without (and you can tell the housekeeping staff at the hotel not to keep putting them on the pillow, too!).

Hotels

If you regularly spend several nights a week away from home and have to rely on hotels or bed-and-breakfast accommodation, try to find a chain or individual establishment that can offer some of the following (remember this is for people who eat in hotels on a daily basis – not necessarily for holidaymakers or weekenders).

Breakfast to go for

- unsweetened, and, better still, freshly pressed, fruit juice
- cereals with no added sugar
- skimmed milk,
- wholemeal toast
- grilled rather than fried breakfast
- a selection of fruit (fresh or dried)
- porridge made with water or low-fat milk and not too much added salt (difficult to find in Scotland!)

Breakfast to bypass

- continental breakfast (e.g. croissant, brioche, *pain au chocolate*)
- Danish pastries
- muffins
- fried breakfast (e.g. sausage, mushrooms, bacon, eggs, fried bread, black pudding and so on)

Working lunches

- Most supermarkets and high street shops offer lower-calorie or lower-fat ranges of sandwiches and lunchtime snack meals. And most have a range of sandwiches of around 300 calories. Also go for sandwiches marked 'No Mayonnaise'.

- Make a regular choice of salad-based snacks or pre-washed and ready-to-eat salad meals.

- If buying a ready-meal to heat up in the office or at home for lunch, check the calorie content on the nutrition panel on the packet. As a rule of thumb, pre-prepared main courses that contain no more than 5g of fat per 100g will be low in calories (as well as fat).

- In some ways, using a sandwich bar where the rolls and sandwiches are made (and the jacket potatoes are filled) to order offers you more control over what you eat. You can stipulate no spread on your bread or no mayonnaise. However, the drawback can be that items such as prawns and tuna are mixed in high-fat (and therefore high-calorie) mayonnaise-based dressings.

- Individual cartons of fruit juice are more nutritious than fruit drinks, which may look the same but contain very little juice and are mainly water and a hefty serving of sugar or artificial sweetener.

- Carbonated drinks such as colas, cordials and squashes, can cause acid erosion of tooth enamel which is far more difficult to treat than dental caries. The main problems are caused if these drinks are taken frequently between meals – something that habitual dieters may tend to do as a substitute for food.

Healthier and leaner meal planning

Many people start planning a meal by first deciding which meat, fish or other protein food to use. A healthier approach is to start by choosing a starchy carbohydrate food on which to base the meal. This is a good idea because these foods should make up the bulk of what you eat. (And they are also low in fat and calories.) Next, choose the vegetable and/or fruit component of the meal, and finally the fish, meat or protein alternative.

Cheer up, you can have chocolate

Although there wasn't that much room for chocolate in the *Fighting Fat, Fighting Fit* Slimming and Healthy Eating Plans, you did see that it was possible to have some chocolate foods – and eat well at the same time.

There is nothing wrong with chocolate and there is no reason why slimmers or anyone else should deny themselves such a fabulous food. Chocolate is far more nutritious than many other types of confectionery – it contains reasonable amounts of iron (so if you allow your children to have sweets, it may be better if they have chocolate).

And if you buy high-quality chocolate, with a cocoa solids content of around 70 per cent, then the taste is so concentrated, sensational and satisfying that a little goes a long way. In fact, studies have shown that a small amount, eaten soon after you fancy it, can head off a serious chocolate binge for so-called chocaholics who are prone to such attacks!

Incidentally, you cannot be addicted to chocolate. Being a chocaholic is a state of mind, not a true physiological addiction.

For most of us, this approach will mean using more bread, cereal, pasta, rice, vegetables and fruit than we do at the moment. And it will also mean regularly including beans, lentils and other pulses, together with nuts.

For tips on using more starchy foods, vegetables and fruit, fish and pulses, and for ways of cutting down on fats, sugar and salt, see Chapter 3.

Healthier cooking methods

Healthier cooking with vegetables and fruit

- Vegetables and fruit are excellent sources of vitamins and minerals. To make sure they remain as nutritious as possible, try to shop for fresh produce every few days and store it in a cool dark place, or in the fridge.
- Prepare vegetables and fruit as close to cooking/eating as possible and avoid soaking them in water for long periods.
- Don't chop fruit or vegetables too small because that exposes more surfaces to nutrient loss.
- Tear the leaves of green leafy vegetables, rather than cutting them with a knife.
- Dress cut vegetables and fruit in lemon juice to prevent vitamin C loss by oxidation.
- Whenever you can, use vegetables unpeeled to retain the vitamins and minerals that are just under the skin, and the fibre in the skin.
- Cook them for the shortest time possible and in the minimum amount of water. Use water in which vegetables have been cooked for soups, sauces and so on because cooking doesn't destroy minerals (as it does vitamins) – they just leach out into the cooking water.
- Add vegetables to boiling water. Better still, steam or microwave them or use a waterless cooker, available from specialist cook shops.
- If you are preparing vegetables for a dish, instead of sautéing them, 'sweat' them in a covered pan where they will cook in their own juices.
- Use puréed vegetables and fruits to thicken savoury and sweet sauces instead of egg yolks, cream or a *roux* (flour and fat paste).

Ways to eat more potatoes

- Instead of having ubiquitous 'chips with everything' for everyday eating: steam, boil or microwave potatoes with the minimum of water.
- Mashed potato makes a much lower-fat topping for 'pies' than pastry and is an excellent starchy-food side dish.
- Baked potatoes are great for lunch, dinner, supper and children's teas.
- Cold potatoes can be made into potato salad (see below). And slimmers will be pleased to hear that cold cooked potatoes are far lower in calories than hot ones because the starches in them become more resistant to digestion once they have been cooked and become cold!

Healthier cooking with potatoes

- Gradually cut down the amount of butter or margarine you add during cooking or at the table. Replace some of these fats with olive oil, but still use the minimum amount. Instead of fat, you can moisten jacket (baked) potatoes with low-fat yoghurt, cottage cheese, fromage frais or lower-fat crème fraîche flavoured with chopped fresh herbs (e.g. parsley, basil, coriander, chervil, fennel, dill) or spices of your choice.
- Mash potatoes with skimmed milk and/or low-fat spread and seasoning or herbs (as above) instead of butter/margarine or cream and salt.
- You can enjoy the colour and flavour of sautéed or 'fried' potatoes by making rosti, a Swiss dish of grated and fried potato cakes that lends itself to cooking with the minimum amount of vegetable oil in a non-stick pan.
- Potato salad tastes just as good made with reduced-calorie mayonnaise or low-fat yoghurt, cottage cheese, fromage frais or lower-fat crème fraîche flavoured with fresh chopped herbs and spices.

Low-fat Home-made Oven Chips

Normal chips contain 350 calories per portion, whereas these low-fat ones only contain 80 calories per portion.

Serves 4

700g (1lb 9oz) potatoes
1 litre (1¾ pints) boiling stock (meat
*   or vegetable)*
2 tablespoons vegetable oil
paprika to taste

Preheat the oven to 220°C/425°F/Gas 7.

Peel the potatoes and cut them into thick chips. Plunge into a saucepan containing the boiling stock and cook for up to 5 minutes, until just tender.

Drain in a colander (reserving the stock for another batch of chips or to use in a soup or sauce). Allow to cool slightly.

Put the oil in a large polythene food bag or plastic food box and carefully toss the chips in the fat. (At this point you can freeze them for later use, once they are cold.)

Transfer the chips to a lightly greased or non-stick baking tray and bake for 10–15 minutes, turning them once or twice, until golden and crisp. If cooking from frozen, allow 15–20 minutes.

Sprinkle with paprika rather than salt, and serve.

Ways to eat more fish

- Make regular use of both white and oily fish.
- Try to eat fish at least twice a week in place of meat, using oily fish on at least one occasion.
- Try making your own fish pies (topped with potato) and fishcakes for a snack meal or light supper – they are both tasty and economical (if you use cheaper types of fish such as coley and mackerel).

- Fish balls make a nice change from fishcakes – mince oily and white fish in a food processor, season and mould into balls, dip in egg wash and roll in flour/breadcrumbs (optional). Bake them on a flat baking sheet or cook them in a tomato sauce.
- Canned fish, such as sardines, pilchards and herring, are cheap and nutritious and a good source of calcium because you can eat the bones. Fish canned in tomato sauce will be lower in calories than fish canned in oil.

Healthier cooking with fish (and poultry)

Steaming retains flavour, colour, shape and nutrients, does not add any calories and is a very successful cooking method for fish and poultry.

Microwaving is also very good for fish and poultry. Cook in a covered microwavable dish with diced vegetables and chopped fresh herbs for extra flavour. There's no need to add fat during cooking.

Poaching is best for delicate white fish (e.g. plaice fillets) or whole oily fish (e.g. salmon, trout and mackerel). Poach them in a light vegetable stock.

Grilling and barbecuing can be done without adding fat to poultry or oily fish.
- Turn frequently during cooking to prevent burning.
- Baste white fish with lemon juice.
- Marinate poultry or meat before cooking to tenderize and reduce cooking time.
- Grill fish fingers and fishcakes rather than frying them.
- If you do fry, use a good-quality non-stick pan so that you don't have to add any fat.

Baking is very good for oily fish steaks (e.g. salmon) and for chunky, firm white fish steaks (e.g. cod and halibut).

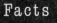

Facts

Fish and chips

This famous British fast food dish is actually very nutritious. However, it is also very high in fat and calories. If you often eat fish and chips, get into the habit of removing some of the batter from the fish because it soaks up lots of fat during cooking. Also, find a chip shop that uses vegetable oil and does not double-cook the chips by reheating once-cooked chips in hot fat. This practice produces poorer quality chips and increases their fat content. When making fish and chips at home, use our Low-fat Home-made Oven Chips recipe (see p. 144).

Healthier cooking with meat (and poultry)

Preparation

- Cut off any visible fat from meat and bacon. Remove the skin from poultry.
- Roast meat without additional fat (see opposite).
- Choose lean or extra-lean mince, which is sometimes labelled 'less than 10 per cent fat'.
- Offal (e.g. liver and kidneys) is a lean and nutritious choice, but it does contain more cholesterol than some other meats. Liver is not recommended during pregnancy because it contains unacceptably high levels of vitamin A. (Although vitamin A is essential for health very high levels can be toxic to unborn babies.)

Grilling

- Grill steaks, chops and other individual cuts of meat on a rack in a grill pan to allow excess fat to drain into the pan to be discarded after cooking.
- There's no need to add fat to any of these items during grilling. Just squeeze over some lemon juice, if necessary.

Roasting

- Place meat on a trivet in a roasting pan so that the fat drains away as the meat cooks. There's no need to add extra fat during cooking – the fat present in the meat will roast it.
- To roast poultry, start it off upside down on a trivet in a roasting pan. (This will allow the fat and juices to drain through the drier breast meat.) Turn for the final half of cooking time to brown. If you think it is in danger of drying out, cover it with a layer of baking paper and/or foil for part of the cooking time.
- Pour the fat away *before* making gravy with the juices. When the gravy is made, let it stand for a few minutes to allow the fat to rise to the top, then spoon it off. Or use a special gravy boat or jug that retains the fat so that it doesn't pour out with the gravy.

Stir-frying

- Small strips of lean meat can be stir-fried with a wide variety of vegetables. This is a very quick method of cooking.
- Thin strips of lean pork, lamb and beef can be marinated before cooking to further reduce cooking time.
- Using a deep wok allows you to use less fat.

Saucy meat cooking

- Instead of making meat the centrepiece of a meal, use smaller quantities in sauces that include lots of vegetables and pulses (such as beans, lentils and chickpeas). You can do this, for example, with pasta sauces and baked pasta dishes (such as lasagne), risotto, paella, pilau, shepherd's pie, casseroles and stews. In casseroles, replace some of the meat with pulses and vegetables (e.g. carrots, swedes, turnips, parsnips and potatoes). Use lean minced, diced or chopped meat for pasta sauces combined with vegetables such as onions, tomatoes, carrots, peppers, courgettes, aubergines, leeks and cauliflower.
- Make stews and casseroles the day before they are needed. Allow them to become cold so that you can remove any fat from the top. Reheat until piping hot before serving.

Ways to eat more nuts and seeds

- Enjoy peanut butter sandwiches, and other nut butters on bread or toast.
- Peanut butter or ground nuts also form the basis of satay sauces and can be used to thicken many spicy oriental dishes and curries.
- Try vegetarian recipes that use nuts as replacements for meat in burgers, loaves, rissoles, cutlets, etc.
- Decorate celebratory cakes and bakes with nuts instead of icings and frostings.
- To make more of seeds, use them as snacks (e.g. pumpkin and sunflower). Add seeds (e.g. poppy, caraway and linseed) to breads and spice cakes. Use seeds (e.g. black or white sesame seeds) as coating instead of breadcrumbs where appropriate.
- Hummus is made from ground chickpeas and tahini (sesame seed paste). Choose a reduced-fat version if you buy it or make your own using the following recipe:

Hummus

You can eat this delicious dip with crudités, crispbread or on hot toast.

200g (7oz) canned chickpeas, drained
1 rounded tablespoon tahini
1 fat garlic clove, peeled
juice of ½ lemon
75 ml (2½fl oz) olive oil or
    80g (3oz) low-fat soft white cheese

Put the chickpeas, tahini, garlic and lemon juice in a food processor and blend them to a paste. You can then thin the paste to the desired consistency by drizzing in the olive oil. Or, for a lower-fat version, blend in the soft, white cheese.

Choosing the right kind of cheese

There is a huge variety of wonderfully tasty and tempting cheeses available today. But it is amazing to think that a matchbox-size piece of Cheddar contains more than 150 calories. The high calorie content is due to the amount of fat in cheese. Here is a quick guide to help you make informed choices when you are buying cheese:

Type	Examples	Calorie percentage from fat
Low-fat	Fromage frais, quark, low-fat soft white cheese	25 per cent or less
Medium-fat	Cottage cheese	35 per cent
	Ricotta and other medium-fat cheeses	25–45 per cent
High-fat	Cheddar and other hard cheeses, blue cheeses, cream cheeses, Edam, Brie Camembert, goat's cheeses. (Edam and Brie are slightly lower in calories than Cheddar-type cheeses)	60 per cent or more

Healthy ways to enjoy cheese

- Use fat-reduced cheese such as half-fat Cheddar.
- Choose a strongly flavoured or mature cheese – especially for cooking, so that a little goes a long way. Tasty cheeses to try include matured Cheddar, Gruyère, Emmental, Parmesan, Pont l'eveque and chevre.
- Replace cream cheese and full-fat soft white cheese with low-fat and medium-fat soft white cheese for sandwich fillings and in recipes.

Slimming tips for cheese

There are some people who never go on a slimming diet, but simply cut out all unnecessary fat over a period of weeks if they need to lose a bit of weight. Not buying cheese for a short while is the best way to do this along with cutting down on butter, margarine and other fats.

If cheese is not sitting in the fridge (and biscuits are not sitting in the tin) then you will automatically eat these high-fat, high-calorie foods less frequently.

Know your creams

There is nothing wrong with eating cream occasionally – strawberries and cream during Wimbledon fortnight are all the more enjoyable when they can be looked forward to as a seasonal treat. Similarly, cream teas taste best when eaten in the garden of a thatched cottage (wasps permitting) on a summer holiday in Devon. It is the habitual eating of fatty foods that causes weight problems. That's why, for everyday eating, lower-fat dairy products are the best option. Here's a quick guide to cream and yoghurt.

Type of cream	Calories per 15ml level tablespoon
Aerosol spray cream	7
Half cream	20
Single, soured or reduced-fat crème fraîche	25
Sterilized canned or whipping cream, whipped	30
Whipping cream	45
Double cream, whipped	50
Double, extra-thick double, or crème fraîche	55
Clotted cream	70

Incidentally, some artificial or non-dairy creams made from vegetable oil contain just as much fat and calories as dairy cream – and they don't taste half as nice as the real thing!

Type of yoghurt	Calories per 125g pot (may vary between brands)
Custard style	165
Bio fruit, Greek or Greek-style	145
Whole-milk fruit	133
Rich and creamy fruit	125
Low-fat fruit	111
French set	100
Whole-milk natural	98
Goat's milk natural	80
Low-fat natural	66
Diet fruit	60

FIGHTING FAT, FIGHTING FIT

AINSLEY'S RECIPES

The recipes are presented in the same order as they appear in the text. There are 16 fabulous slimming plan dishes and 20 delicious healthy eating plan recipes, including pasta, salads, curries, stir-fries, soups, snacks, kebabs, easy family meals and dinner party dishes.

Main Meal Recipes

Fuzzyless Jerk Chicken

Jerk chicken is a really tasty way to enjoy chicken without adding lots of fat. Be careful with the habaneros or Scotch bonnet chillies. They are the hottest in the world – so you may want to adjust the amount you use.

Serves 6

225g (8oz) onions, peeled and quartered

2 habaneros or Scotch bonnet chillies, halved and seeded

50g (1³⁄₄oz) fresh root ginger, peeled and roughly chopped

½ teaspoon ground allspice

leaves from 15g (½oz) fresh thyme sprigs

1 teaspoon freshly ground black pepper

125ml (4fl oz) white wine vinegar

125ml (4fl oz) dark soy sauce

6 part-boned chicken breasts

Put all the ingredients, except the chicken, in a food processor and whizz until smooth.

Put the chicken in a large, shallow non-metallic dish, pour over the sauce, cover and leave to marinate in the fridge for 24 hours, turning the chicken every now and then.

Grill or barbecue the chicken breasts under or over a medium heat for 25–30 minutes, basting now and then with the leftover sauce. As it cooks, the thickened sauce will go quite black in places, but as it falls off it will leave behind a really well-flavoured, crisp skin, with lovely moist, tender meat underneath.

- This recipe includes the chicken skin, but to further cut down on fat discard the skin from poultry and game.

Ainsley's Ultimate Creole Cabbage Salad

Far more colourful and tastier than standard coleslaw, this recipe uses only a minimum of mayonnaise so it is low in fat and high in flavour.

Serves 6

280g (10oz) white cabbage, cored and very thinly shredded

2 celery sticks, thinly sliced

1 green pepper, seeded and very thinly sliced

4 spring onions, trimmed and thinly sliced

½ tablespoon Dijon mustard

1 teaspoon creamed horseradish

1 teaspoon (5ml) Tabasco sauce

1 tablespoon red wine vinegar

2 tablespoons olive oil

2 tablespoons mayonnaise

salt (optional) and freshly ground black pepper

2 tablespoons chopped fresh dill

a pinch of cayenne pepper

Mix the cabbage, celery, green pepper and spring onions together in a large bowl.

Mix the mustard, creamed horseradish, Tabasco and vinegar in a small bowl and then gradually whisk in the oil. Stir in the mayonnaise and season well.

Stir the dressing and chopped dill into the vegetables just before serving so that the cabbage stays nice and crunchy. Sprinkle with the cayenne pepper and serve.

Peppy's Jamaican Rice and Peas

In this traditional Jamaican dish, 'peas' means red kidney beans, pigeon peas or black-eyed beans, not the green garden peas. This must be one of the most delicious ways to eat more pulses and the dish keeps well in the fridge for several days (if there is any left!). Make it with brown rice, if you prefer, and reduce the quantities of butter and creamed coconut if you want to cut down on saturated fats.

Serves 8

1 onion or 3 spring onions, trimmed and finely chopped
1 tablespoon sunflower oil
25g (1oz) butter
2 garlic cloves, peeled and finely chopped
1 red chilli, seeded and very finely chopped
450g (1lb) long-grain rice

2 sprigs of fresh thyme
7.5cm (3 inch) piece of cinnamon stick (optional)
400g (14oz) can red kidney beans, black-eyed beans or pigeon peas, drained
125g (4½oz) creamed coconut, coarsely grated
½ tsp salt (optional)

Fry the onion or spring onions in the oil and butter for 2 minutes, then add the garlic and chilli and fry for another 2 minutes over a medium heat.

Stir in the rice and thyme, and cinnamon stick if using, until everything is well coated in the oil.

Pour in the beans or peas, add the grated creamed coconut and stir until the coconut has dissolved.

Then stir in 1 litre (1¾ pints) hot water, with the salt if using. Bring to the boil, cover and cook over a low heat for 25–30 minutes (up to 45 minutes if using brown rice).

Remove from the heat and set aside, undisturbed, for 5 minutes.

Remove the thyme and cinnamon, season to taste, and serve.

Melintzanosalata with Cherry Tomato Sticks

This wonderful (unpronounceable!) Greek dish encapsulates the taste of Mediterranean cooking, demonstrating how delicious healthy eating can be. If you do not want to go to the trouble of making the tomato sticks you could offer a range of crudités instead.

Serves 6

1 large aubergine
juice of ½ lemon
3–4 tablespoons extra virgin olive oil
a good pinch of ground cumin
1 garlic clove, peeled and crushed
1 tablespoon chopped fresh flatleaf
   parsley
2 tablespoons Greek natural yoghurt
salt (optional) and freshly ground
   black pepper

FOR THE TOMATO STICKS:
450g (1lb) cherry tomatoes
4 garlic cloves, peeled and thinly sliced
24 small bay leaves
4 tablespoon olive oil
12 × 15cm (6 inch) bamboo skewers,
   soaked in cold water for 30 minutes

Pierce the aubergine near the stem with a fork to prevent it popping during cooking.

Place it under a medium-hot grill, or over a medium-hot barbecue, and cook for 20 minutes, turning now and then until the skin is really black and starting to blister and the flesh feels tender in the centre.

Meanwhile, thread three tomatoes on to each skewer, alternating them with a slice of garlic and a bay leaf.

Cut the aubergine in half lengthways and scoop out the flesh. Mash to a rough purée, then mix in the lemon juice.

Very gradually whisk in the olive oil – the mixture will thicken slightly. Stir in the ground cumin, garlic, parsley and yoghurt, and season to taste. Spoon into one or more bowls. Just before serving, drizzle with any olive oil left over from basting the tomatoes.

Brush the cherry tomato sticks with the olive oil. Place them under a medium-hot grill, or over a medium-hot barbecue, and cook for 4–5 minutes, turning every now and then, until just soft and the skins have split. Season and serve with the dip and Garlic Pitta Fingers.

Garlic Pitta Fingers

Made in a matter of minutes, these are deliciously buttery without being excessively fatty. To speed up the process, you can melt the butter in the microwave. But be careful, as it takes only seconds.

Serves 6

50g (1³/₄oz) unsalted butter, melted
2 garlic cloves, peeled and very finely
  chopped

2 tablespoons chopped fresh parsley
6 sesame or white pitta breads

Put the butter in a small pan and heat gently until melted. Add the garlic and parsley and just heat through. Set aside to allow the flavours to combine. Lightly slash the pittas on one side and place, cut side up, under a grill or to one side of a barbecue and cook for 1 minute until lightly toasted.

Turn the pittas over and spoon over the garlic butter. Cook for another 1–2 minutes until sizzling.

Lift the pittas on to a board and cut into thick fingers. Serve warm.

Sweet Chilli King Prawns

These are expensive, but they are a special treat for slimmers who need to concentrate on flavour and quality of food rather than quantity! Prawns are low in fat and packed with protein.

Serves 6

36 raw freshwater king prawns or
   72 headless raw tiger prawns
3 tablespoons vegetable oil
1 tablespoon clear honey
1 tablespoon Tabasco sauce
finely grated zest and juice of ½ lime

3–4 garlic cloves, peeled and crushed
salt (optional) and freshly ground
   black pepper to taste
6–12 × 25cm (10 inch) thin metal
   skewers

Peel the prawns, leaving the last tail section in place. Make a shallow cut along the curved back of each one and lift out the dark, thread-like intestine.

Mix the rest of the ingredients together in a large bowl. Stir the prawns into the mixture and leave them to marinate in the fridge for up to 2 hours.

Thread the prawns on to the skewers. If you are using king prawns you will be able to thread six prawns on to one skewer for each person. If you are using tiger prawns you will need to do two skewers per person.

Grill or barbecue the prawns under or over a medium heat for 3–4 minutes, turning them now and then until they are firm and opaque. Eat them while they are still hot.

Cor! Puy Lentil, Red Onion and Sun-dried Tomato Salad

This is one of the most delicious ways to enjoy lentils and relatively easy to make. If you do not have time to cook the lentils, you can use ready-cooked canned ones.

Serves 8

225g (8oz) Puy lentils, picked over to remove stones
1 fresh bay leaf
1 teaspoon red wine vinegar
2 garlic cloves, peeled and left whole
a pinch of caster sugar
salt (optional) and freshly ground black pepper
1 large red onion, peeled and finely chopped

50g (1¾oz) sun-dried tomatoes in oil, drained and chopped
1–2 tablespoons balsamic (or other) vinegar
4 tablespoons extra virgin olive oil
115g (4oz) goat's cheese or feta cheese, crumbled
3 tablespoons chopped fresh flatleaf parsley

Put the lentils in a pan with the bay leaf, vinegar, one whole garlic clove, sugar and a little salt, if using, and pepper. Cover with 1.2 litres (2 pints) cold water, bring to the boil and leave to simmer for about 25 minutes, until the lentils are just tender but still holding their shape.

Drain the lentils well, discarding the bay leaf and whole garlic clove. Tip them into a salad bowl and leave to go cold.

Finely chop the remaining garlic clove and stir into the lentils with the rest of the ingredients. Season to taste and chill for 2 hours before serving to let the flavours soak into the lentils.

Crispy Baton Bacon Potato Cakes

This recipe shows how a little mature cheese can go a long way in terms of adding flavour – the mustard accentuates the flavour of the cheese.

Serves 4

500g (1lb 2oz) floury potatoes, peeled and diced

1 tablespoon olive oil

4 rashers smoked lean back bacon, cut into 2cm (³/4 inch) wide strips

50g (1³/4oz) mature Cheddar, grated

1 teaspoon English mustard

4 salad onions, trimmed and finely chopped

50g (1³/4oz) plain flour

salt (optional) and freshly ground black pepper

1 teaspoon butter or vegetable oil

Cook the potatoes in boiling water for 10–15 minutes until tender. Heat the olive oil in a large frying pan and cook the bacon strips for 3–4 minutes until crisp and well browned.

Drain the potatoes and mash well; stir in the crispy bacon, Cheddar, mustard, onions, plain flour, salt, if using, and plenty of pepper. Shape the mixture into eight even-sized cakes.

Heat the butter or vegetable oil in the bacon pan and gently cook the potato cakes for 3–4 minutes on each side until well browned.

Teasing Turkey Pitta Pockets

This is a great way to fill lean meat full of flavour.

Serves 4

1 tablespoon vegetable oil
1 teaspoon butter
1 onion, peeled and thinly sliced
2 garlic cloves, peeled and finely
    chopped
50g (1¾oz) fresh white breadcrumbs
6 fresh sage leaves, finely chopped
grated rind and juice of 1 lemon
½–1 teaspoon Cajun seasoning or
    mild chilli powder
200g (7oz) cooked turkey, cut into
    1cm (½ inch) strips

salt (optional) and freshly ground
    black pepper
4 pitta breads

TO SERVE:
shredded iceberg or cos lettuce
sliced red onion
4 tablespoons Greek yoghurt
wedges of lemon (optional)

Heat the oil and butter in a large frying pan and cook the onion and garlic for 3–4 minutes until softened and golden. Stir in the breadcrumbs, sage, lemon rind, Cajun seasoning or chilli powder, and turkey, and stir-fry for 2–3 minutes, until the breadcrumbs begin to brown. Add the lemon juice and season to taste.

Make a slit in the side of each pitta. Mix together the lettuce and red onion and pack into the bottom of each pitta pocket. Pile in the turkey mixture and top with a dollop of yoghurt, and, if you like, a squeeze of lemon juice.

Fab Haddie and Gooey Egg

A super light and easy supper. After you've finished the slimming plan you can continue to use this recipe – serve it with a chunk of your favourite flavoured bread to dip into the runny yolk, plus some broccoli.

Serves 4

1 tablespoon olive oil
1 onion, peeled and sliced
400g (14oz) canned chopped
  tomatoes
2 tablespoons chopped fresh parsley,
  plus extra to garnish

salt (optional) and freshly ground
  black pepper
4 × 115g (4oz) pieces smoked
  haddock, skinned
2 tablespoons white wine vinegar
4 eggs

Heat the oil in a large frying pan and cook the onion for 4–5 minutes until golden. Stir in the tomatoes and parsley and season to taste. Place the fish pieces on top, cover and simmer for about 8 minutes until the fish is cooked.

Meanwhile, add the vinegar to a medium pan of boiling water. Then lower the heat slightly and swirl the water round with a spoon. Crack two of the eggs into two separate cups, then gently slide both eggs into the swirling water. Cook for 2–3 minutes until the white is set but the yolk is still runny (see note below). Remove and drain with a slotted spoon; keep warm. Repeat with the other two eggs.

Spoon the sauce and fish on to serving plates. Top each with an egg, sprinkle with parsley and season with pepper.

- Do not serve undercooked eggs to young children, pregnant women or other 'at risk' groups because of the risk of salmonella poisoning.

Chargrilled Pineapple Chicken Kiss-Kiss

A fabulous combination of meat and fruit – far tastier than all those high-fat breaded chicken, fried chicken and chicken-ready meals ...

Serves 6

6 large boneless chicken breasts,
    unskinned
225g (8oz) prepared fresh
    pineapple or pineapple canned
    in natural juice
2–3 spring onions, trimmed and
    thinly sliced

salt (optional) and freshly ground
    black pepper
60g (2¼oz) caster sugar
a pinch of chilli powder
6 small, thin metal skewers, or
    cocktail sticks soaked in cold water
    for 30 minutes

Cut a small shallow pocket into the side of the thickest part of each chicken breast.

Drain the pineapple and reserve the juice. Finely chop the pineapple and mix with the spring onions and a little salt, if using, and pepper. Spoon the mixture into each pocket and secure with a skewer or cocktail stick.

Mix the reserved pineapple juice and sugar together in a small pan and leave over a low heat until the sugar has dissolved. Bring the mixture to the boil and boil vigorously until it is syrupy and reduced to about 4 tablespoons. Stir in the chilli powder.

Grill or barbecue the chicken under or over a medium heat for about 10 minutes, turning now and then, until it is about half-cooked. Then brush over some of the pineapple glaze and continue to cook for another 10 minutes, turning and brushing the chicken with more glaze until it is cooked through and the skin is nice and golden.

Wicked Wine-steamed Mussels

A dish that looks and tastes really sophisticated, yet is simple to do and really low in calories. Mussels are naturally quite salty – so there is no need to add any salt during cooking.

Serves 2

150ml (5fl oz) dry white wine
1 small onion, peeled and very finely
  chopped
2 garlic cloves, peeled and thinly sliced
1 red chilli, seeded and finely chopped,
  or a pinch of dried chilli flakes

1kg (2¼lb) scrubbed live mussels
freshly ground black pepper
a handful of fresh parsley, roughly
  chopped

Pour the wine into a large saucepan with a close-fitting lid. Add the onion, garlic and chilli and bring to the boil. Simmer for 5 minutes, until the onion is tender.

Meanwhile, check the mussels, discarding any that remain open when tapped sharply with a knife (if they do not close, they are dead and should not be eaten).

Add the mussels to the pan with a good grinding of black pepper, cover and steam for 3–5 minutes, shaking the pan occasionally, until all the shells have just opened. Discard any that do not open after cooking.

Sprinkle the parsley over and ladle the mussels and wine juices into large bowls.

Cheesy Cherry Tom Potato Omelette

Eggs are so convenient and they team up well with vegetables. Try this with green vegetables for a change, instead of potatoes. The natural creaminess of an omelette also means you will not miss having butter with your bread.

Serves 2

50g (1³/₄oz) Edam or mozzarella, grated

4 cherry tomatoes, quartered

4 small cooked new potatoes, sliced

1 tablespoon snipped fresh chives

4 eggs

a little salt (optional) and freshly ground black pepper

1 teaspoon butter

¹/₂ teaspoon olive oil

Mix together the grated cheese, tomato quarters, potato slices and snipped chives. Beat together the eggs and a little seasoning in a separate bowl.

Melt the butter and oil in a 23–25cm (9–10 inch) frying pan, then pour in the beaten egg. As the omelette cooks, use a fork to gather the set egg into the centre of the pan so the runny egg can run to the edge and cook. Continue to cook over a low heat for several minutes until just set.

Preheat the grill to high. Tilt the pan, then use a spatula to roll up the omelette. Carefully transfer the omelette to a warm heat-proof plate, ensuring that the join is underneath.

Cut a slit along the top and spoon in the tomato and chive mixture. Place under the grill for 1 minute to melt the cheese and warm the filling. Season and serve hot.

Down-in-a-Flash Pumpkin and Potato Soup

Pumpkins are packed with beta–carotene, one of those valuable and protective antioxidants. Their flesh is rich and creamy and makes a super smooth soup (or you can have it chunky). This is a brilliant way to enjoy pumpkins, especially if you have not tried them before.

Serves 4

50g (1³/₄oz) butter
3 garlic cloves, peeled and crushed
2 medium onions, peeled and sliced
1 tablespoon medium-strength curry powder
750g (1½lb) pumpkin, peeled, seeded and cut into 2.5cm (1 inch) cubes
750g (1½lb) potatoes, peeled and cut into 2.5cm (1 inch) cubes
400g (14oz) can chopped tomatoes

2 tablespoons chopped fresh coriander
½ teaspoon cayenne pepper
250ml (9fl oz) coconut milk
1.2 litres (2 pints) vegetable stock
salt (optional) and freshly ground black pepper
a pinch of grated nutmeg
150ml (5fl oz) carton natural yoghurt (optional)

Melt the butter in a large saucepan, then fry the garlic and onions for 1 minute without letting them colour. Add the curry powder and stir for 30 seconds, then add the cubed pumpkin and potatoes. Continue to fry and stir for about 5 minutes.

Now add the tomatoes, coriander and cayenne pepper, and stir in the coconut milk and vegetable stock. Bring to the boil, cover and simmer for 35–40 minutes. Remove from the heat and leave to cool slightly.

Liquidize the soup, then return to a clean pan for reheating. If you like your soup chunky, use a potato masher to break up some of the pieces instead of liquidizing. Season to taste, add the nutmeg, and serve with a dollop of natural yoghurt, if liked.

Simply Smokin' Paella

Lean smoked ham gives this paella a distinctive flavour. Paella is a great dish to master, because you can ring the changes with seemingly endless combinations of lean meat, fish and vegetables.

Serves 4

2 tablespoons vegetable oil
1 onion, peeled and sliced
1 red pepper, seeded and sliced
1 garlic clove, peeled and crushed
200g (7oz) long-grain rice
175g (6oz) smoked ham, roughly diced
850ml (1½ pints) chicken or vegetable stock

½ teaspoon each paprika and ground turmeric (or a few strands of saffron, if you have them)
175g (6oz) large prawns, thawed if frozen
115g (4oz) frozen peas
salt (optional) and freshly ground black pepper

Heat the oil in a large frying pan and cook the onion for 3–4 minutes until softened and golden. Add the red pepper, garlic and rice and stir-fry for 1 minute. Add the ham, stock, paprika and turmeric (or saffron), bring to the boil and simmer for 12 minutes.

Stir in the prawns and peas and cook for a further 3–4 minutes, until the rice and vegetables are tender. Season to taste, then serve immediately.

Plantain, Pumpkin and Chickpea Curry

Plantains, which look like large bananas, are a starchy vegetable. They can be cooked in different ways, depending on ripeness. Yellow ones are suitable for quick frying or curries, like this one; and yellow-black plantains are good for desserts. Green ones are best for plantain chips and stews.

Serves 4

4 tablespoons vegetable oil
1 teaspoon whole cumin seeds
1 dried red chilli pepper, seeded and
    crushed
1 onion, peeled and sliced
2 garlic cloves, peeled and chopped
2.5cm (1 inch) piece of root ginger,
    peeled and grated
1 teaspoon ground coriander
1/4 teaspoon ground turmeric
5cm (2 inch) stick of cinnamon or
    1/2 teaspoon ground cinnamon
450g (1lb) pumpkin, peeled, halved,
    seeded and cut into roughly 2.5cm
    (1 inch) cubes

280g (10oz) plantain, peeled and
    cut into cubes
400g (14oz) can chopped tomatoes
225g (8oz) canned or cooked
    chickpeas, drained
2 tablespoons medium-hot curry paste
300ml (10fl oz) stock
1 tablespoon chopped fresh coriander,
    plus extra for garnish
salt (optional) and freshly ground
    black pepper

TO SERVE:
1 banana
1 tablespoon lemon juice

Heat the oil in a deep pan. Fry the cumin seeds for 5 seconds, then add the chilli, followed by the onion and garlic. Fry for 1 minute, then add the remaining spices. Stir and cook for another minute.

Add the pumpkin and plantain, and mix until everything is well coated with the spices, and the vegetables begin to turn slightly brown. Add the tomatoes, chickpeas, curry paste and vegetable stock and stir well. Bring to the boil, cover and simmer for 20–25 minutes or until the pumpkin is tender and the sauce is nice and rich. Stir in the fresh coriander, and season to taste.

Peel and slice the banana and toss it in the lemon juice. Serve the curry in a bowl and top with sliced banana and chopped coriander.

Spicy, Sunny Savoy Cabbage with Bacon and Ginger

If you tend to be reluctant to 'eat up your greens', this recipe will show you just how versatile and delicious the humble cabbage can be.

Serves 4

3 tablespoons olive oil

50g (1¾oz) unsalted butter

2.5cm (1 inch) piece of root ginger, peeled and cut into fine strips

1 small red chilli, seeded and sliced into rounds

3 rashers rindless smoked lean back bacon, cut into fine strips

150g (5½oz) carrots, peeled and cut into matchsticks

280g (10oz) Savoy or white cabbage, cored and finely sliced

3 tablespoons soy sauce

2 tablespoons clear honey

salt (optional) and freshly ground black pepper

Heat the oil and butter in a wok or large frying pan. Add the ginger and chilli and stir-fry for 30 seconds. Add the bacon and continue to stir over a high heat for 30 seconds. Then add the carrots and cook for 1 minute.

Add the cabbage, mix well and cook for 2–3 minutes. Pour over the soy sauce and honey and season to taste. Serve hot.

Lunch Recipes

Baked Potato, Pepper and Onion Frittata

This Italian version of a Spanish omelette wins more healthy eating points because it contains more fresh vegetables than its Iberian counterpart.

Serves 4

280g (10oz) potatoes, peeled and cut into 1cm (½ inch) cubes
4 tablespoons olive oil
1 large onion, peeled and finely sliced
½ green pepper, seeded and sliced
½ red pepper, seeded and sliced
1 green chilli, seeded and sliced
5 large eggs, beaten
250g (9oz) ricotta
55g (2oz) freshly grated Parmesan
salt (optional) and freshly ground black pepper

Preheat the oven to 180°C/Gas 4/fan oven 160°C, parboil the potatoes for 5 minutes and drain.

Heat the oil in a frying pan. When hot, add the potatoes and gently fry until golden, then remove with a slotted spoon and drain on kitchen paper.

In the same pan, fry the onion until lightly golden. Add the peppers and chilli, fry for 1 minute, remove with a slotted spoon and drain on kitchen paper.

When well-drained, mix the potatoes, onion, peppers and chilli with the beaten egg, then mix in the ricotta and Parmesan and season to taste.

Pour into a well-buttered, spring-form tin or an oven-proof buttered frying pan and bake for 35–40 minutes until the centre is firm and the top is golden brown. (You can always brown it a bit more under the grill.) Loosen the frittata around the edges, turn out on to a plate, cool slightly, cut into wedges and serve.

Chicken Show-Stopper Stir-Fry

Cook the rice or noodles beforehand because, once you have prepared the ingredients, this dish is ready in minutes. It is another happy combination of low-fat poultry with lots of lovely vegetables.

Serves 4

1 celery stick
1 carrot, peeled
½ red pepper
½ green pepper
1 small head broccoli
4 baby sweetcorn
6 button mushrooms
2 boneless chicken breasts, cut into
  strips 1cm (½ inch) wide
  and 7.5cm (3 inches) long
2 tablespoons soy sauce
1 tablespoon sesame oil

2 tablespoons vegetable oil
3 spring onions, trimmed and sliced
  at an angle
1 garlic clove, peeled and chopped
2.5cm (1 inch) piece of root ginger,
  peeled and finely chopped
80g (3oz) beansprouts
2 tablespoons clear honey
2 tablespoons hoisin sauce (Chinese
  barbecue sauce)
freshly ground black pepper

Cut the celery, carrot, peppers, broccoli, baby sweetcorn and mushrooms horizontally into slices or lengthways into batons.

Mix the chicken with the soy sauce and sesame oil in a bowl. Heat a wok or large frying pan, add the vegetable oil and swirl it around so the wok is well coated. Then add the chicken and stir-fry for 2–3 minutes. Remove with a slotted spoon and keep warm.

Throw the spring onions, garlic and ginger into the wok and fry for 30 seconds. Then add all the vegetables, except the beansprouts, and continue to stir-fry over a high heat until tender but still crisp.

Now add the beansprouts, chicken, honey, hoisin sauce and 2 tablespoons water. Toss over the heat for 3–4 minutes, season with pepper and serve.

Main Meal Recipes

Munchie Mustard Chicken Escalopes

Make the mountain of salad as high as you like.

Serves 4

4 large chicken breasts
4 tablespoons olive oil
2–3 tablespoons Dijon mustard
1 garlic clove, peeled and crushed
salt (optional) and freshly ground
  black pepper
1 ciabatta loaf
1 teaspoon lemon juice
snipped fresh chives, to garnish

FOR THE SALAD:

50g (1³⁄₄oz) baby spinach leaves
1 bunch watercress, large stalks
  removed
¹⁄₂ small head radicchio lettuce
4 tablespoons mayonnaise
1 tablespoon Dijon mustard

Put each chicken breast between two large sheets of clingfilm and beat out gently with a rolling pin until it is about 5mm (¹⁄₄ inch) thick.

Mix 3 tablespoons of the oil with the mustard and the crushed garlic. Brush some of this mixture over both sides of the chicken and season.

For the salad, place the prepared leaves in a bowl and lightly toss. Mix the mayonnaise with the mustard and set aside with the salad.

Cut the ciabatta in half lengthways as if you were going to make a sandwich, and then across, making four chunky pieces. Place cut side up under a preheated grill or cut side down on a barbecue and lightly toast.

Grill the chicken under a medium-hot grill or over a barbecue for about 3 minutes each side, until golden on the outside and juicy in the centre. Chicken is cooked when the juices run clear, not pink.

Whisk the rest of the olive oil, lemon juice and seasoning into the remaining mustard mixture. Add to the salad and toss together lightly.

Place a piece of ciabatta on each plate and spread with a little mustard mayonnaise. Sprinkle over a few leaves, then put a piece of chicken on top, followed by more leaves. Add another dollop of the mustard mayonnaise and sprinkle with a few snipped chives. Serve at once.

Moroccan Spiced Lamb Kebabs

This is another great way to cook meat, without adding any fat, so that it's full of flavour. Harissa is a fiery red chilli paste from northern Africa. It can be found in supermarkets, but you can replace it with minced red chilli if you wish.

Serves 4

900g (2lb) boned shoulder or
    leg of lamb
3 tablespoons olive oil
2 tablespoons lemon juice
1 teaspoon ground cumin
1 teaspoon ground coriander
½ teaspoon ground turmeric
½ tablespoon paprika

1 garlic clove, peeled and crushed
1 tablespoon harissa
salt (optional) and freshly ground
    black pepper
1 small red onion
1 small lemon
4 × 30cm (12 inch) flat metal
    skewers

Trim any excess fat off the outside of the lamb and then cut into 5cm (2 inch) chunks. Place in a bowl with the olive oil, lemon juice, spices, garlic, harissa and some seasoning and mix well. Cover and leave to marinate at room temperature for 2 hours, or overnight in the fridge.

Peel the onion, leaving the root end intact, and then cut into eight wedges, so that the slices of onion stay together at the root. Cut the lemon into eight wedges.

Thread the lamb chunks, and lemon and onion wedges alternately on to the skewers and grill under a medium-hot grill, or over medium-hot coals, for 10–15 minutes. Turn now and then, until they are nicely browned on the outside, but still pink in the centre.

Spicy Casablanca Couscous

A wonderfully zestful combination of couscous, fresh herbs, spices and pine nuts – a delicious accompaniment to any grilled fish or meats. Try making your own version with nuts, as an innovative way to make your life nuttier!

Serves 10

3 tablespoons olive oil

1 garlic clove, peeled and very finely chopped

1 teaspoon ground cumin

1 teaspoon ground coriander

1 teaspoon paprika

350ml (12fl oz) chicken or vegetable stock

a good pinch of saffron strands

6 spring onions, trimmed and thinly sliced

225g (8oz) couscous

2 red chillies, seeded and very finely chopped

50g (1³⁄₄oz) pine nuts, toasted

coarsely grated zest and juice of 1 lemon

1¹⁄₂ tablespoons chopped fresh coriander

1¹⁄₂ tablespoons chopped fresh mint

1¹⁄₂ tablespoons chopped fresh parsley

Heat 2 tablespoons of the oil in a large pan. Add the garlic, cumin, coriander and paprika and fry for 1 minute, stirring.

Add the stock and saffron and bring to the boil. Add the spring onions and then pour in the couscous in a steady stream and stir once.

Cover the pan with a tight-fitting lid, remove from the heat and set aside for 5 minutes, to allow the grains to swell and absorb the liquid.

If you are serving this warm, stir in the rest of the oil and the remaining ingredients now. Otherwise, leave the couscous to cool and chill in the fridge for 1 hour before adding all the other ingredients.

Sally's Salmon Steaks with Fresh Basil Sauce

Unlike pesto, which is quite high in calories and fat because it is made with Parmesan and pine nuts, this fresh-tasting sauce is just made with lots of basil, lemon juice and olive oil and goes perfectly with barbecued salmon.

Serves 4

4 × 200g (7oz) salmon steaks
1 tablespoon olive oil
salt (optional) and freshly ground
   black pepper

FOR THE FRESH BASIL SAUCE:
40g (1½oz) fresh basil
1 tablespoon freshly squeezed lemon juice
salt (optional) and freshly ground
   black pepper
6 tablespoons olive oil

First make the sauce. Set aside four sprigs of basil for a garnish. Remove any large stalks from the remainder and put in a food processor, with the lemon juice and a little seasoning.

Switch on the machine and, once the basil has blended to a paste, very slowly pour in the olive oil. Taste, adjust the seasoning and set the sauce on one side.

Brush the salmon steaks on both sides with a little oil and season. Grill under a medium-hot grill, or barbecue over medium-hot coals, for 4–5 minutes on each side, until golden on the outside but still moist and juicy in the centre. Garnish with the basil sprigs and serve with the fresh basil sauce.

Speckled-eye Squash Stew

This stew positively oozes goodness, yet it's easy to make and tastes terrific. The beauty of a one-pot meal is not just less washing up, but also the fact that all the vitamins and minerals are kept in the sauce – and eaten.

Serves 3

2 tablespoons olive oil
½ teaspoon cumin seeds
½ teaspoon mustard seeds
1 onion, peeled and chopped
1 garlic clove, finely chopped
1 red chilli, seeded and sliced
450g (1lb) potatoes, scrubbed and
    roughly chopped
2 tablespoons curry paste
600ml (1 pint) vegetable stock

450g (1lb) squash, butternut, pumpkin
    or kabocha, peeled and roughly diced
400g (14oz) can black-eyed beans,
    drained
2 tomatoes, each cut into 6 wedges
salt (optional) and freshly ground
    black pepper
2 tablespoons chopped fresh coriander or
    parsley to garnish
lemon wedges to serve

Heat the olive oil in a large pan, add the cumin and mustard seeds and cook for 1 minute. When they begin to splutter and pop, add the onion, garlic and chilli and cook for 3–4 minutes until softened.

Stir in the potatoes and cook for 3 minutes. Add the curry paste and vegetable stock, bring to the boil and simmer for 5 minutes. Add the squash or pumpkin, and simmer for a further 15 minutes until the vegetables are tender. Add the black-eyed beans and tomatoes and continue to cook for 2–3 minutes. Season to taste.

Divide the stew between individual dishes, sprinkle over the coriander or parsley and serve with lemon wedges.

Tossed Beansprout Prawn Noodles

Frozen prawns are fine for this recipe, but if you're making it for a special occasion you could use large tiger prawns. Noodles have all the same health benefits as pasta – combined with prawns and vegetables they provide a well-balanced meal. Oyster sauce is available from most supermarkets.

Serves 2

175g (6oz) medium egg noodles
2 tablespoons vegetable oil
1 garlic clove, peeled and chopped, or
   1 teaspoon garlic purée
1 tablespoon chopped fresh coriander
   or parsley
6 salad onions, trimmed and
   diagonally sliced
1 red chilli, seeded and chopped

115g (4oz) mushrooms (oyster,
   chestnut or button), sliced
115g (4oz) large cooked peeled
   prawns
3 tablespoons oyster sauce
1 tablespoon fresh lime juice
2 teaspoons caster sugar
115g (4oz) beansprouts
coriander or parsley sprigs to garnish

Cook the noodles in boiling water for 4 minutes, or according to the packet instructions, then drain well.

Meanwhile, heat the vegetable oil in a frying pan and stir-fry the garlic, chopped coriander or parsley, salad onion slices and chilli for 1 minute. Add the mushrooms and prawns and stir-fry for a further 1 minute.

Stir in 120ml (4fl oz) water, the oyster sauce, lime juice and sugar. Cook briefly to heat through and reduce slightly. Stir in the noodles and beansprouts and heat through. Toss, garnish with a few sprigs of coriander or parsley, and serve.

Cod Kebabs with Aztec Salsa

A beautiful quick supper that makes the most of fresh ingredients. If you like your salsa with a kick, add one small, fresh, seeded, chopped chilli. The capers are quite salty, so you may prefer not to add any more salt when seasoning.

Serves 3

450g (1lb) thick cod fillets, skinned and cubed

grated zest of 1 lime

juice of 2 limes

3 tablespoons olive oil

salt (optional) and freshly ground black pepper

3 tomatoes, seeded and chopped

1 small red onion, peeled and finely chopped

1 tablespoon chopped fresh parsley or coriander

1 tablespoon drained capers

1 courgette, diagonally sliced

225g (8oz) tagliatelle

6 fine metal skewers, or bamboo skewers soaked in cold water for 30 minutes

Mix together the cubed cod, lime zest, half the lime juice and 1 tablespoon of the oil. Season with pepper and set aside for 5 minutes.

Mix the tomato flesh, onion, 1 tablespoon of the oil, the parsley or coriander, capers and the remaining lime juice.

Preheat the grill to high. Thread the cod cubes and courgette slices on to the skewers, season and grill for 8–10 minutes, turning once, until tender and golden.

Meanwhile, cook the tagliatelle in a large pan of boiling water, salted if you wish, according to the packet instructions. Drain, then toss with the remaining oil (optional). Fork some tagliatelle into the centre of each plate, top with two kebabs and spoon over some salsa.

Iced Fresh Fruit Platter with Passionfruit Cream

Leave the skin on the fruit for extra 'grip' when dipping it into the cream and to boost vitamin and fibre intake. It's also more colourful.

Serves 8

1 papaya
1 mango
1 small pineapple
4 kiwi fruit
1 small Galia or Charentais melon

FOR THE PASSIONFRUIT CREAM:
4 passionfruit
150ml (5fl oz) double cream
finely grated zest of ½ small orange
2 tablespoons icing sugar
2 tablespoons orange juice
5 tablespoons Greek-style yoghurt

For the passionfruit cream, cut the passionfruit in half and scoop out the pulp into a bowl.

Whip the cream, orange zest and icing sugar into soft peaks and then gradually whisk in the orange juice, yoghurt and passionfruit pulp so that the mixture remains softly whipped. Spoon the mixture into a small serving bowl, cover and chill in the fridge.

Cut the fruits into one-portion pieces. Place on a tray and cover. Put in the fridge until just before you are ready to serve.

Arrange the chilled prepared fruits attractively on a large serving platter around the bowl of cream.

Char Sui Lettuce Rolls

Char Sui is the Chinese name for that infamous 'red' roast pork dish found in almost every Chinese restaurant. Here, it is carved into very thin slices, and rolled up inside lettuce leaves with crunchy spring onions, cucumber and plum sauce. Add as much salad garnish as you like.

Serves 4

2 × 450g (1lb) pork fillets
5cm (2 inch) piece of fresh root ginger, peeled
1 large garlic clove, peeled and crushed
2 tablespoons hoisin sauce
2 tablespoons dark soy sauce
2 teaspoons light soft brown sugar
1 teaspoon Chinese five-spice powder
2 tablespoons (30ml) vegetable oil

4–6 drops red food colouring (optional)
2 tablespoons clear honey

TO SERVE:
½ cucumber
6 spring onions, trimmed
1 large iceberg lettuce, broken into leaves
175ml (6fl oz) Chinese plum sauce

Trim any fat and gristle off the outside of the pork fillets.

Finely grate the ginger and squeeze out the juice into a shallow non-metallic dish. Stir in the rest of the ingredients. Add the pork fillets and turn them over in the mixture until they are well coated. Cover and set aside for at least 2 hours.

Cut the cucumber in half lengthways and scoop out the seeds with a teaspoon. Cut into thin strips about 7.5cm (3 inches) long. Halve the spring onions and cut lengthways into very thin shreds. Arrange on a serving plate in separate piles, along with the lettuce leaves and a small bowl of the plum sauce.

Grill or barbecue the pork fillets under or over a medium heat for about 20 minutes, turning now and then and basting with the leftover marinade, until the juices run clear when the meat is pierced.

Transfer the pork to a board, carve it into very thin slices and then pile it on to a warmed serving plate. To eat, flatten a lettuce leaf, put a little plum sauce down the centre, then a line of cucumber strips, shredded spring onion and sliced pork. Roll up the lettuce leaf parcel and eat!

Sinhalese Pasta

A brilliant meal that's ready in 20 minutes! Try using spaghetti or
noodles for a change.

Serves 2

450g (1lb) linguine pasta
salt (optional)
½ teaspoon oil
6 tablespoons olive oil
½ small onion, peeled and finely
    chopped
1 garlic clove, peeled and crushed
1 tablespoon curry powder

1 tablespoon chopped fresh coriander
1 tablespoon chopped fresh mint
1 tablespoon chopped fresh parsley
225g (8oz) peeled prawns
zest and juice of 1 lemon
salt (optional) and freshly ground
    black pepper

Cook the pasta in a large pan of water, salted if you wish, adding the
½ teaspoon oil to prevent sticking. When the pasta is *al dente* (tender but
still offering some resistance when bitten), remove from the heat
and drain. Heat the olive oil in a large frying pan or wok, add the onion
and garlic and fry without allowing them to colour. Add the curry
powder and stir-fry for 20 seconds, then throw in all the herbs, prawns
and lemon zest. Toss to heat through, then add the lemon juice.

Lightly season, add the cooked pasta, toss again, and serve.

Cor!! Coriander Lemon Chicken

A really tasty and refreshing chicken dish that goes excellently with the Cool Carrot, Cumin and Lemon Salad (see opposite).

Serves 4

1.5kg (3lb) chicken, cut into 7.5cm
  (3 inch) pieces
salt (optional) and freshly ground
  black pepper
3 garlic cloves, peeled and chopped
2 tablespoons lemon juice
2 tablespoons ground coriander
50g (1³/₄oz) butter
2 tablespoons olive oil

TO GARNISH:
sprigs of fresh coriander or roughly
  chopped coriander
lemon wedges

Preheat the oven to 190°C/Gas 5/fan oven 170°C. Season the chicken, rub in the garlic, lemon juice and ground coriander, then marinate in a covered non-metallic dish for 2–3 hours or overnight in the fridge.

Heat the butter and oil in a frying pan and brown the chicken over a high heat. Remove and put into an ovenproof dish, pour the butter and oil from the pan over the top, then bake for 1–1¼ hours until cooked through. If you like it browner on top, pop it under the grill for 1–2 minutes.

Serve garnished with sprigs of coriander or sprinkled with chopped coriander, and lemon wedges.

Cool Carrot, Cumin and Lemon Salad

A simple salad that can be put together in not much more than
10 minutes, proving that fresh vegetables are nature's convenience food.

Serves 6

750g (1lb 10oz) carrots
½ teaspoon salt (optional)
4 tablespoons sunflower oil

1 tablespoon cumin seeds
1 tablespoon black mustard seeds
4 tablespoons lemon juice

Top and tail and then peel the carrots. Either coarsely grate them, or cut
them lengthways, with a potato peeler, into long ribbons. Put the carrot
in a bowl and toss with the salt, if using.

Heat the oil in a small pan. When it is quite hot, toss in the cumin and
mustard seeds and leave them to sizzle for a few seconds.

As soon as the mustard seeds begin to pop, pour the mixture over the
carrots in the bowl and toss together with the lemon juice.

Grilled Tuna with Green Lentil Salad

Tuna is the fillet steak of the fish world. It should be cooked lightly, as overcooking will dry it out. You can even eat it slightly under-done.

Canned pulses usually contain added salt. If you prefer to avoid this, use dried lentils. To give them flavour without adding salt, cook them in chicken stock with a few vegetables (e.g. carrots, celery, onion, garlic) and a bay leaf.

Serves 2

425g (15oz) can green lentils
2 plum tomatoes, finely chopped
55g (2oz) diced mixed peppers (red, green or yellow)
1 chilli, seeded and finely chopped
1 spring onion, trimmed and finely chopped
2 tablespoons soy sauce
1 tablespoon white wine vinegar

3 tablespoons olive oil
1 tablespoon mixed chopped fresh herbs (e.g. coriander, basil and parsley)
salt (optional) and freshly ground black pepper
2 × 175g (6oz) fresh tuna fish steaks
sprigs of fresh coriander to garnish

Put the lentils in a saucepan and warm slightly. Remove from the heat and drain. If using dried lentils, cook them as described in the introduction, then drain them and remove the vegetables and the bay leaf. Place in a large bowl, then add the chopped tomatoes, peppers, chilli and spring onion. Now add the soy sauce, vinegar, 2 tablespoons of the olive oil and the fresh herbs. Season and mix well and set aside.

Heat a cast-iron ridged grill pan until hot. Season the tuna steaks and brush with the remaining olive oil. Grill for 2–3 minutes on each side, depending on their thickness. Place a mound of lentil salad in the middle of each plate, carve a tuna steak at an angle and arrange on top of the salad with a garnish of fresh coriander.

Red Stripe Linguine with Chestnut Mushrooms and Basil

If we haven't told you already, pasta is high in fibre and low in fat. It is at the heart of the healthy traditional Mediterranean diet and recipes like this show how tasty it can be without the addition of butter or cream.

Serves 1

150g (5oz) linguine pasta
salt (optional)
½ teaspoon vegetable oil
3 tablespoons olive oil
1 garlic clove, peeled and crushed
115g (4oz) chestnut or brown
  mushrooms, sliced

2 sun-dried tomatoes, cut into strips,
  or 1 fresh tomato, seeded and cut
  into strips
4 basil leaves, torn into small pieces
freshly ground black pepper
freshly grated Parmesan

Cook the pasta in a pan of water, salted if you wish, adding the ½ teaspoon oil. When *al dente* (tender but still offering some resistance to the teeth when bitten), remove from the heat and drain.

Heat the olive oil in a frying pan, add the garlic and, 10 seconds later, the mushrooms. Fry for 1–2 minutes, until the mushrooms start to sweat. Add the sun-dried or fresh tomato and basil leaves and toss.

Add the drained pasta, season, toss again and serve with a sprinkling of Parmesan.

Pinky Grapefruit, Prawn and Green Avocado Salad

A winning, highly nutritious combination of fruit and shellfish that also looks and tastes stunning.

Serves 4

2 pink grapefruit
2 medium avocados
200g (7oz) packet mixed lettuce leaves
115g (4oz) cooked peeled prawns
½ red pepper, seeded and cut into
  fine strips

FOR THE DRESSING:
6 tablespoons light olive oil
1 tablespoon white wine vinegar
¼ teaspoon ground allspice
1 teaspoon chopped fresh
  coriander

Peel and carefully segment each grapefruit over a bowl to catch the juice, then squeeze the juice out from the core and skin. Put the juice to one side.

Cut the avocados in half, remove the stones and peel off the skin. Cut each half into three slices lengthways. Place the lettuce leaves on four serving plates, arrange three slices of avocado on top of each serving, and divide the grapefruit segments between them. Scatter over the prawns and the strips of red pepper.

To make the dressing, vigorously shake or whisk the grapefruit juice, oil, vinegar, allspice and coriander until well mixed. Drizzle over the salad before serving.

Crunchy Cod and Mash

This snappy dish is ready in a flash (15 minutes is pretty flashy!). It's such a tasty way to serve fish that you could also make it with unsmoked white fish for a change.

Serves 4

15g (½oz) butter, plus extra for greasing

4 × 150g (5oz) smoked cod fillets, skinned

salt (optional) and freshly ground black pepper

6 salad onions

4 tomatoes, sliced

8 black olives, pitted and chopped

2 tablespoons olive oil

3 tablespoons torn fresh basil leaves

25g (1oz) fresh white breadcrumbs

700g (1lb 9oz) potatoes, peeled and chopped

4–5 tablespoons milk

Preheat the oven to 200°C/Gas 6/fan oven 180°C.

Put the fish in a lightly buttered ovenproof dish and season. Chop the white parts from the onions, slice and scatter over the cod. Arrange the tomatoes on top of the fish and scatter over the olives. Drizzle over half the oil and sprinkle with half the basil. Toss the breadcrumbs with the remaining basil, season and scatter over the fish. Drizzle over the remaining oil and bake for 15 minutes until the fish is cooked.

Meanwhile, cook the potatoes in a pan of boiling, salted (optional), water for 10–15 minutes. Drain well, then add the milk and mash to a soft consistency. Put the mash to one side of the pan, add the butter and heat. Finely chop the green parts of the onions, add to the pan and fry briefly. Stir the onions into the mash and season.

Divide the onion mash between the serving plates and place the cod on top. Spoon around the fish juices and serve.

Smoked Bacon, Creamy Tomatoes, Peas and Penne Pasta

Peas are a great source of vitamin C, and they go well in lots of pasta dishes. Using smoked bacon means you will not need salt for seasoning – if you find smoked bacon too salty use unsmoked (green) bacon.

Serves 2

2 tablespoons olive oil

4 rashers lean smoked rindless bacon, cut into strips

2 shallots, peeled and finely chopped

80g (3oz) frozen garden peas

1 teaspoon chopped fresh tarragon

85ml (3fl oz) dry white wine

280g (10oz) passata (sieved tomatoes)

150ml (5fl oz) double cream or crème fraîche

280g (10oz) fresh or dried penne pasta

½ teaspoon oil

freshly ground black pepper

freshly grated Parmesan

Heat the oil in a pan and fry the bacon until lightly brown, then add the shallots, and fry for a further minute. Add the peas, tarragon and white wine, and bring to the boil for 2 minutes. When it starts to bubble stir in the passata.

Reduce the heat, stir in the cream or crème fraîche, cover and simmer for 8–10 minutes.

Meanwhile, cook the pasta in a large pan of water, salted if you wish, adding ½ teaspoon oil. When *al dente* (tender but still offering some resistance to the teeth when bitten), remove from the heat and drain.

Taste the sauce and season with black pepper. Mix in the cooked pasta and serve with the Parmesan.

Superb Mackerel with Chilli and Herbs

Mackerel is packed full of vitamins and has all the health benefits of oily fish. It is excellent value for money and is available all year round. This is a great recipe to get you into the habit of eating oily fish at least once a week.

Serves 4

4 × 280g (10oz) whole mackerel,
gutted and cleaned
55g (2oz) fresh mixed herbs (e.g.
chives, dill, parsley and tarragon),
chopped
2 red chillis, seeded and finely chopped

1 tablespoon sesame oil
2 tablespoons olive oil
2 tablespoons soy sauce
salt (optional) and freshly ground
black pepper
oil for frying

Make three 5mm (¼ inch) deep slashes across each fish, then repeat in the opposite direction. Reserve half the herbs and put the rest inside the fish. Transfer to a shallow dish.

Mix together the reserved herbs, chillis, sesame and olive oils, soy sauce and seasoning. Spoon over the fish, working it into the slashes. Cover and chill for 2 hours.

Heat the oil in a large frying pan. Cook the fish on the uncut side for 4 minutes. Then place under a medium grill, cut side up, for 4–6 minutes until crisp.

Index